# Eating
# THIN
## *for*
# LIFE

# Eating
# THIN
## *for*
# LIFE

*Food Secrets & Recipes from*
*People Who Have Lost Weight*
*& Kept It Off*

## Anne M. Fletcher,
### M.S., R.D.

#### With a Foreword by Graham Kerr

*A Companion Book to*

## Thin *for* Life

*10 Keys to Success from*
*People Who Have Lost Weight & Kept It Off*

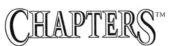

Chapters Publishing Ltd., Shelburne, Vermont 05482

Published by
Chapters Publishing Ltd.,
2085 Shelburne Road, Shelburne, VT 05482

"Are You Kidding Yourself" adapted from "What's in a Portion?" *Tufts University Diet & Nutrition Letter*, Volume 12, No. 7, September 1994.

Chicken Wild Rice Soup and Heartland Corn Chowder adapted from *Healthy Exchanges Food Newsletter*, Volume IV, Issue 1, January 1995, by JoAnna M. Lund, Healthy Exchanges, DeWitt, Iowa.

Polynesian Carrot Salad and Sweet and Sour Pork adapted from *HELP: Healthy Exchanges Lifetime Plan* by JoAnna M. Lund with Barbara Alpert, G.P. Putnam's Sons, New York, 1996.

Party Turkey Tetrazzini, Denver Pizza and Southern Banana-Butterscotch Cream Pie adapted from *Healthy Exchanges Cookbook* by JoAnna M. Lund, G.P. Putnam's Sons, New York, 1995.

Luscious Black Bean Soup, Fat-Free Creamy Italian Dressing, Heavenly Brownies, Rich Chocolate Frosting and Chocolate Upside-Down Cake adapted from *Lean and Lovin' It* by Don Mauer, Chapters Publishing Ltd., Shelburne, Vermont, 1996.

Middle Eastern Chicken, Grilled Honey-Dijon Pork and Pirate's Pie adapted from *Sensibly Thin: Low-Fat Living and Cooking, Volume II*, by Sam Eukel, Sensibly Thin, Fargo, North Dakota, 1994.

Library of Congress Cataloging-in-Publication Information
Fletcher, Anne M.
    Eating thin for life: food secrets & recipes from people who have lost weight
and kept it off / Anne M. Fletcher ; cover illustration by Kathy Warinner.
        p.      cm.
    Includes index.
    ISBN 1-57630-020-X (hardcover)
    1. Weight Loss. 2. Weight loss—Case studies. 3. Reducing diets—
Recipes. I. Title.
    RM222.2.F5357  1996
    613.2'5—dc20                                    96-27632

Printed and bound in Canada by Best Book Manufacturers, Inc.

Designed by Susan McClellan

10 9 8 7 6 5 4 3 2 1

FOR JULIA AND JULIA,
MY MOTHER AND MY DAUGHTER

# Author's Note

A S WITH ALL DIETS AND WEIGHT-LOSS PROGRAMS, you should
obtain your physician's permission and seek his or her supervision before and while following the meal plans, recipes and/or
advice in *Eating Thin for Life*. This is particularly important if you
have a medical problem, such as diabetes, high blood pressure or heart
disease. A registered dietitian's counsel is advised as well. If you have
psychological distress, such as serious depression or high stress in
your life, you should see a psychologist or a psychiatrist before following *Eating Thin for Life*'s recommendations. The author and publisher disclaim any liability arising directly or indirectly from the use
of *Eating Thin for Life*.

All masters in *Eating Thin for Life* have given their permission to
share information about their weight and eating habits. Some of the
masters' names have been changed to protect their privacy. Sometimes, the masters' remarks were edited slightly for clarity. In Chapter Six, "Meals from the Masters," some meals were adapted. When
necessary, recipes were adapted.

# ACKNOWLEDGMENTS

**W**ITHOUT THE MASTERS OF WEIGHT CONTROL, this book would never be. I first want to thank the hundreds of men and women who have shared their weight-loss success stories and their wonderful recipes. I am grateful, as well, for the help of the weight-loss organizations, friends and colleagues who helped me recruit the masters.

My deep appreciation goes to Carla Chesley for her skills in refining and testing the masters' recipes. Thanks, too, to my recipe tasters: the Stolp family, the Robbins-Black family, the fine staff at Chesley, Kroon, Chambers & Ingman law firm. I also want to express my gratitude to both Mary Stadick and Tammi Hancock, R.D., for their expert technical assistance with research, and to nutritionist Mary Jane Laus of the Massachusetts Nutrition Data Bank at the University of Massachusetts, Amherst, who did the nutrition analyses for the recipes.

It almost goes without saying that I am indebted to Rux Martin, my editor, Barry Estabrook, Chapters' editor-in-chief, and Chris Tomasino, my agent, for their support and belief in my work. And I continually appreciate professional input from my friends Larry Lindner and Gail Zyla at the *Tufts University Diet & Nutrition Letter*.

Finally, I thank the behind-the-scenes people who helped to make my life manageable while I was writing *Eating Thin for Life*; namely, Beverly Rauchman, Barb Brockhaus, Nedra Tweit, Maggie Stolp, Alex Filipovitch, Inez Thomas and Cindy Balk. Finally, I appreciate beyond all measure the support and patience of my own kin, Steve, Wes, Ty and little Julia.

# CONTENTS

# Foreword

T HESE DAYS, WE'RE SO BOMBARDED with scientific data, national surveys and opinion polls that it's easy to forget the value of personal experiences. In fact, should one be brave enough to venture an opinion based on a personal story, it's often cynically dismissed as "anecdotal." It's almost as though great stories of individual success are irrelevant in the mind of a "demographically inclined" scientist.

Now, mind you, I'm just as thrilled as anyone else to get my hands on new data and the latest studies, especially those having to do with food, nutrition and lifestyle change. Those statistics, however, are a bit dismal right now. They show that America spends close to $38 billion every year on weight-loss methods—but as a nation, we're still gaining weight!

It all seems quite hopeless until we set aside the headlines, forget the advertising claims and begin to read about individual stories of successful weight loss.

Those are the stories that Anne Fletcher has gathered here, along with some solid research and open-minded reporting. These moving stories from people just like you and me give us all hope that healthy, lasting change might be more within our reach than we ever thought possible. The personal testimonials will not only give you practical guidance for dealing with your own weight control, they will renew your faith in the power of individuals to take charge of their health.

As both a research "subject" and a reader of Anne's previous book, *Thin for Life*, I can attest to her mastery of this complex issue. Her philosophy, writing and interviews have been valued guideposts to me as I have pursued my own research.

I strongly suspect that Anne is deeply motivated by what I call a C3 syndrome. A C3 person is, first of all, *committed* to serve people. Second, a C3 person has a genuine sense of *compassion*—in this case, for those who have struggled, often unsuccessfully, with weight control. Lastly, and as a direct result of their compassion, C3 people are fueled with a desire to be *consistent*.

One of the greatest motivational speakers of all time—a C3 person if ever there was one—was once asked, "What is the greatest lifestyle rule?"

He responded, "Love God with all your heart, soul, mind and strength." Then, without pause, he went on to say, "And the second is similar . . . love your neighbor as you would love yourself."

Including yourself in your list of people you love does you no harm and, in my experience, is essential if you are going to master your weight.

When my oldest daughter, Tessa, was 12, she asked me why I worked so hard (those were the "Galloping Gourmet" recording days). I replied that when the 650th show was finished, our family would sail away on our sailboat for a year to spend more time together. "Wouldn't it be sad," she said, "if, when you finished, you had a checkup, and because you smoke so much . . . they found cancer . . . and you died . . ." (she is very dramatic) "and you never got to fulfill your dreams!"

Tessa was my messenger; I stopped smoking on that day in 1970.

And now I'm telling you that within these pages, you may hear *your* messenger. Read, make notes, ask questions. I am sure there are at least a dozen bright ideas and scores of tested recipes that will help you. Find those that fit your personality and your lifestyle . . . then, find in your heart the will to be consistent and apply those principles to your day-to-day life.

Best wishes on your journey to change; I wish you lasting success. And, when you reach your goal, you should speak out confidently about your victory . . . and simply smile quietly when someone refers to it as "anecdotal."

# Introduction

D O YOU WANT TO LOSE WEIGHT? Do you want to keep it off for good? Then you'll want to turn to the *real* experts at weight control: the very people who have done it. That's what I did. For a number of years now, I've been closely studying "masters" of weight control—people who have lost at least 20 pounds and have kept them off for 3 or more years.

I focus on the success stories because I'm tired of hearing about all the people who lose weight and gain it back. I'm certain there are far more slimmed-down people out there than we've been led to believe—I've single-handedly found hundreds of them.

It's been said that 95 percent of all dieters gain back the weight they worked so hard to lose. When I hear that statistic, I want to scream. Who made it up? According to renowned obesity experts Kelly Brownell, Ph.D., and Judith Rodin, Ph.D., the failure figure has its roots in a single survey conducted in a hospital nutrition clinic in 1959. More recent statistics on relapse come from people who participate in studies conducted at universities. But individuals who are drawn to research-based programs appear to have tougher, hard-core weight problems than do overweight people in the general population, who eventually lose weight on their own, through self-help groups or with the help of commercial weight-loss programs. *I maintain, as do a number of other experts, that the chance of success at permanent weight loss is greater than we've been led to believe.*

Several years ago, I located 160 masters who, instead of remaining heavy all their lives or boomeranging up and down, succeeded in coming to grips with their weight problems permanently, keeping off, on average, a surprisingly high 63 pounds. My previous book, *Thin for Life: 10 Keys to Success from People Who Have Lost Weight & Kept It Off,* reveals the many things these masters have in common. In the first place, after years of struggling—gaining, losing, then gaining again—they reach a critical turning point where they finally believe in their own abilities to solve their problems. (Many had been heavy since childhood and didn't lose weight once and for all until they were in their 40s, 50s and even older.) They stop seeing themselves as failures and begin to view themselves as individuals who can take responsibility for their weight, recognizing that no one else can do it for them.

I discovered that one of the masters' most powerful techniques is nipping small gains in the bud. That is, nearly all have a maximum upper limit—usually no more than 5 to 10 pounds above their goal—and they are adamant about not exceeding it. When they hit that line, a plan of action goes into effect. The masters also use some powerful psychological strategies, such as engaging in the art of positive self-talk. That is, they counter destructive thoughts that can trigger overeating with productive words of encouragement. Instead of turning to food when they're bored, upset, lonely or stressed out, the masters have learned to cope more effectively.

NOT SURPRISINGLY, MOST OF THEM EXERCISE. But although physical activity is an integral part of their lives, most are not fanatical about it. Perhaps best of all, somewhere along the route to becoming successful maintainers, many masters realize they aren't getting enough out of life and are spurred to develop more balanced, fulfilled and happy existences. In essence, I found that the masters are people who take control so their weight will stop controlling them.

Clearly, in order to keep off all that weight, the masters have made major changes in their food habits. Many acquire a taste for low-fat eating and experiment with and learn to enjoy new foods.

After I finished writing *Thin for Life*, the masters' relationships with food continued to fascinate me. There were so many more questions I wanted to ask:

• Once they've lost the weight, do they have to keep track of calories so they won't get heavy again?

• Do they feel like they're forever on a diet, or do they really enjoy food?

• How do they stay motivated after the thrill of losing weight is gone—when everyone stops noticing?

• Do they actually *like* low-fat foods or feel that they *have to* eat them?

• Do they eat fast food or allow themselves hot-fudge sundaes? How do they handle cravings?

• How often do they eat? Are they grazers, or are they three-meal-a-day eaters?

• Do they have to discipline themselves to stop eating, or have they learned to recognize when they're full?

• How do they deal with family members who seem to be able to eat all they want or who could care less about eating healthfully? Do they make separate meals for themselves, or does the whole family have to change?

• What do they do about pushy friends and relatives who urge them to "try just one slice" of cheesecake or "just one more" serving of mashed potatoes?

• How do they survive rocky times like quitting smoking, premenstrual days, pregnancy and even the loss of loved ones without gaining weight back?

• Do they "let loose" in restaurants, at parties or when on vacation?

To FIND THE ANSWERS, I went back to the original masters and also recruited many new ones. This time, I located 208 slimmed-down people, most of whom far exceed my definition of a master of weight control. *The average weight loss of the masters I spoke with is 64 pounds. In fact, 30 masters have kept off 100 pounds or more!*

Some of the masters have been thin for so long that their friends never knew they were once overweight. Consider Nancy K., who's been a master for 10 years. She's moved to a new location since she lost her 64 pounds and says, "Most people don't believe I was ever heavy—

so I often have to prove it with pictures!" *Indeed, the average length of time the masters have kept off 20-plus pounds is more than 10 years.*

Who are the masters? They come from all walks of life—they're secretaries, teachers, scientists, homemakers, physicians, lawyers, nurses, computer specialists and retirees. Some are friends of friends and relatives of friends. Many responded to newspaper announcements and flyers I circulated across the country. In addition, a number of masters were referred to me by weight-control organizations, such as TOPS (Take Off Pounds Sensibly), Diet Center, Overeaters Anonymous, Optifast, Health Management Resources, Weight Watchers and Nutri/System.

I N EATING THIN FOR LIFE, the masters share the intimate secrets of their food lives, revealing how they ate when they were heavy and how they converted to a new way of eating. They explain how they made the often shaky transition from actively losing weight—or dieting—to the keeping-it-off-forever state of maintenance. Exciting common threads emerged. While many people imagine that slimmed-down individuals must exist in Spartan desperation, *the masters are living happy food lives.* When I asked them, "Do you enjoy food?" the overwhelming majority answered "Yes."

Take the case of 154-pound Bob W., whose weight topped out at 400 pounds in eighth grade. He says, "My eating plan gives me health, freedom, vitality and enjoyment—what a deal!" And at 2,000 calories per day (which Bob knows he consumes, because he keeps records), he is certainly not starving!

Bob is not alone—more than 9 out of 10 masters answered "No" to the question, "Do you feel like you're dieting?" In fact, "I eat whatever I want" was one of the most common responses when the masters were asked to describe their eating habits.

But how did they get to this point? That's what *Eating Thin for Life* is all about: how the masters learned to eat what they want and want what they eat. They describe how they motivated themselves to change their eating habits in the first place *and* how they continue to stay motivated.

WHEN IT COMES TO EATING THE WAY THEY DO to keep the weight off, each of the masters does it his or her own way. For instance, Judy C., who has kept off 112 pounds for 18 years, deviates from the three-meal-a-day routine of most masters. She tries to eat two normal meals daily and to cut off her eating by 4 p.m. She says, "I eat like a king for breakfast, a queen for lunch and a pauper for dinner." Ron K. (61 pounds, 7 years)* is unique in his choice of baked potatoes as a mainstay of his diet. He eats a minimum of two per day, with a variety of toppings. He even eats a baked potato before going out to dinner, to stave off his hunger so that he can order sensibly. JoAnn L. (74 pounds, 26 years) rarely uses reduced-fat desserts, as do many masters, but allows herself a regular sweet treat each day. She also has red meat more frequently than most masters. *It's important to pick and choose what works for you from the "secrets" of the masters to find a way of eating to suit your lifestyle, food preferences, special needs and problems.*

In "Part I: Food Secrets of the Masters," the masters share their strategies for long-term success—in the kitchen, at the table, in restaurants, at parties and in challenging situations. "Part II: Meals from the Masters" provides a weight-loss plan based on the masters' favorite breakfasts, lunches, dinners and snacks—21 days of ideas for lively, varied meals that you can mix and match so you can shed pounds without struggling with complicated "exchanges" or fancy recipes. Finally, in "Part III: Eating Thin for Life Recipes," the masters share more than 100 of their favorite recipes for breads, breakfasts, soups, sandwiches, main dishes, side dishes and desserts—easy low-fat dishes that they cook again and again.

Whether you want to lose 10 pounds, 50 pounds or more, *Eating Thin for Life* will show you how to lose weight—and keep it off—without suffering or denying yourself what you really like to eat. *If the masters did it, you can do it too.*

---

* *When two numbers are given after a person's name, the first refers to the number of pounds the person has lost and the second refers to the length of time that person has been a master of weight control.*

# PART I

# FOOD SECRETS
## *of the*
# MASTERS

CHAPTER ONE

Food Secret #1:

# Want to Be Thin More Than You Want to Eat the "Wrong" Foods

"**H**OW WOULD YOU DESCRIBE YOUR FOOD HABITS?" That's what I asked each master to tell me in 25 words or less. As I studied their responses, it struck me: The real issue isn't so much "How do you eat?" as *"How do you get yourself to keep doing what you know you should do?"* You see, the masters pretty much eat the way we all know we should eat to lose weight and keep it off. They go easy on added fats like butter, margarine, oil and mayonnaise and often use low-fat or fat-free versions of these foods. They tend to turn to chicken and fish in place of red meat. They eat lots of fruits and vegetables. They steer clear of greasy and fast foods. They use skim and part-skim dairy products. No big surprises here.

But how come they can do it when so many people can't?

Kay D. answers this question for me in a metaphorical way when she states, *"You have to want to be thin more than you want to eat the 'wrong' foods."* She is describing a crucial shift in thinking—a flipping of the switch, if you will—from seeing what you need to do to be thin as an asset rather than a liability.

In order to change your food habits permanently, you must reach a critical turning point where you feel that the benefits of being thinner overshadow the costs—the effort involved. *First, you have to change your mind-set . . . then your palate will follow.*

# Kay D.'s Story

I T'S HARD TO BELIEVE that petite, attractive, confident 5'3" Kay D. once weighed more than 200 pounds and was in an unhappy marriage in which she repeatedly heard, "Look at you. No one would ever want you. You'll never amount to anything." As she explains, "I hated myself, I hated what I looked like. Food was the only thing that was enjoyable." Today, Kay weighs 114—down 111 pounds from her all-time high. Not only that, but she has fulfilled her lifelong dream of running her own business and can boast, "I just can't say enough for losing weight and what it's done for me and how I feel about life."

Kay, who is 47, exudes happiness. It was a long time coming. Her weight problem had its beginnings around the time of her first marriage, which took place about a year after she graduated from high school. From there, her weight escalated with three difficult pregnancies, each of which required a lot of bed rest. "I would try to lose weight, but it didn't work or I would get pregnant again." After her third child was born in 1977, she found herself at more than 200 pounds. When the baby was 3 months old, Kay and her husband split up. "At that point," she recalls, "I had very low self-esteem and began eating myself into oblivion and gained some more weight. The more I gained, the more introverted I became."

She remarried but soon found herself in a relationship with a man who was both physically and verbally abusive. Somehow, she managed to go to Weight Watchers and lose 40 pounds. "But as soon as I got it off, I went straight back to my old habits, and within six months, it was back on again. I wanted to eat more than I wanted to be thin!"

All told, Kay figures that she tried to lose weight at least 10 to 15 times before she was finally successful. A spiral of self-change began for Kay when, after five years of marriage, her abusive husband left her for another woman. "My kids were growing up, and I started looking within myself. I knew I wanted something out of life, but I didn't know exactly who I was." Two people—one a counselor, the other a new man in her life—convinced her that "you can be whatever you want to be." She started asking herself, "Where am I going to be in 10 years? Do I want to be this size for the rest of my life?" When she looked in the mirror, she didn't like what she saw. "When I put a belt on and would try to sit down in a skirt, the fat roll would hang over the waistband. I wanted something better for myself. I decided this was my last chance."

In April 1992, she went to her local Nutri/System office, where she was told it would cost her, upfront, a dollar a pound to lose the 78 pounds she then wanted to shed. At the time, she weighed 193. She admits, "I had one foot in the door and one foot out. Then I thought, 'Well, maybe if I put the money down, I will be more inclined to hang in there.' Everything I started, I never finished, and for once in my life, I wanted to finish something. I wanted to stand back and be proud of something that I had done for myself."

Kay told her two junk-food-loving teenage sons that things would have to change. "In the past when I went on diets, I didn't do anything about my cooking. This time, I felt that I had to be stronger and in control, because I didn't want the situation to control me." Her children were unimpressed: "Yeah, right, Mom. How long is it going to last this time?" At first, they tried to tempt Kay, but as they saw her progress, they became supportive.

Kay stayed with her diet even when the Nutri/System office in her area closed and she had to drive three hours, round-trip, to the nearest one, which was in another state. She told herself, "I've made this commitment," and she was "determined that nothing was going to stand in my way.

"The more I lost, the better I felt about myself. I was like the caterpillar that went in and the butterfly that came out. Instead of rewarding myself with something good to eat when I lost weight, I'd go to the store and try on clothes to see what sizes were starting to fit." Soon, she became inspired to start walking short distances. "I put on headphones, and I would think about motivational things, like, 'When I lose this weight, here's what I'm going to do . . . ' "

Even before she reached her goal, Kay had developed the confidence to begin doing things that were on her "someday" list. She became licensed to start her own medical-training business. Today, she holds a daytime job as a computer specialist and runs her business at night.

She stuck with her diet for seven months, achieving her goal in October 1992. "The day I weighed in and reached my goal," she recalls, "was one of the scariest days of my life." She had to go off the program's prepackaged foods, which had been the mainstay of her diet, and start making her own food choices. For the next year, she kept regular appointments with her weight-loss counselor. (She still goes back to weigh in about every three months.) She spent time studying the maintenance food book she had been given, which taught her how to "count" various foods and explained how many calories and grams of fat she should have. Her maintenance daily calorie level was about 1,800, and she ate a balanced diet that provided roughly 30 fat grams (15 percent of calories from fat) a day. She felt the calorie level was a little high, so today, she consumes between 1,500 and 1,700 calories a day.

Simply stated, Kay just did her homework: "I planned my meals, counted calories and fat grams, kept track of food groups and weighed and measured just about everything. Before I would eat anything or fix anything or buy anything prepackaged, I'd try to look it up." She attempted to model her meals after those she had been given while dieting. She also kept things simple—for instance, a skinless chicken breast, rice and a vegetable. Kay explains: "It all started coming together—stuff I didn't even know I was learning as I was losing the weight. For instance, I realized that basically, I could eat anything I want to eat—in moderation. If I still wanted to have a peanut butter cookie, I had to compensate by eating less of something else." After about six months, she no longer needed to use the food guide book. "I knew the foods I could eat and which foods were right and which ones weren't."

When she was heavy, she admits that before she had even finished one meal, she'd be thinking, "Okay, what am I going to eat for the next one?" She says, "There were times when I wouldn't have any cash, and I'd go through the family's coats saying, 'I've got to have some French fries,' or 'I've got to have this milkshake.' I used to hide foods so the kids wouldn't eat them. I would eat a whole bag of little peanut butter cups. When the kids would walk into the room, I'd stop chewing, because I knew they'd say, 'Mom, you always say you're going to lose weight.' "

Now, Kay usually starts her day with a large banana and bowl of high-fiber cereal, such as Fiber One, topping it with skim milk. Sometimes, she has fat-free waffles or half a bagel, and on weekends, she treats herself to pancakes, which she eats in a restaurant. (To save calories, she brings her own sugar-free syrup.) Most days, her big meal is eaten at lunchtime. She prepares it at home the night before, so she can just warm it in the microwave at work. Lately, her lunch has been 2½ ounces of pasta, which she weighs before cooking, topped with several slices of fat-free cheese and a 14½-ounce can of unsalted tomatoes—or zucchini, broccoli and mushrooms—which she chops, then seasons with hot sauce, oregano and freshly ground black pepper. It all adds up to a lot of food, she notes, and people say to her, "How in the world are you going to eat all that?"

A year or two into maintenance, Kay gradually lost her taste for meat and became a vegetarian. She quips, "If it has a face, I won't eat it." She is not hungry for a big meal at suppertime, so every evening, her "meal" is a bowlful (1 to 1½ cups) of Healthy Choice low-fat ice cream, which she selects from the four or five flavors she keeps on hand. She always uses the same small bowl so she knows how much ice cream she's getting, but she piles it high so it feels as though it's a lot. Then she eats it with a baby spoon to make it last longer.

Kay uses no oil, butter or margarine and hasn't had any fried foods in four years. Instead, she uses nonstick cooking sprays (like Pam) and fat-free margarine. Her milk, yogurt and cheese are all fat-free. At restaurants, she might order grilled vegetables over rice or pasta. If she can't find anything healthful on the menu, she'll order a large salad with low-calorie or fat-free dressing on the side. When restaurant portions are generous, she eats half of what she's served and takes the rest home in a doggy bag.

I ask Kay how she keeps at it. "It's what matters most to you—your taste buds or looking in the mirror," she replies. "And looking in the mirror matters more to me than 5 to 10 minutes of chewing stuff like French fries and fried chicken. My desire to remain thin out-weighs my desire for the wrong foods. That is my key." Sometimes at night, after she's had ice cream, she finds herself thinking of eating again. She stops herself with, "I want something else more than I want to go to that refrigerator."

# Flipping the Switch

WHEN I ASK CONNYE Z., who has kept 33 pounds off for 6 years, how she sticks with her routine of planning meals, eating low-fat foods, paying attention to calories and exercising diligently, she replies, "For me, it is the joy of being thin. It matters more than eating dessert every day at lunch as opposed to eating fruit." Then there's 6-year master Ted H., who explains why he's now willing to snack on fruits and vegetables rather than on his old favorites of bread, butter, peanut butter and cheese. Having kept off 142 pounds, he has multiple reasons: "I feel better physically. My clothes fit better. Women find me attractive. I am healthier. I don't have to dread go-ing out in public. Nothing tastes as good as being thin feels. What more motivation do I need?"

So how do you flip the switch to get to the point where your de-sire to be thin outweighs your desire to engage in the behaviors that keep you from being thin? How do you get yourself to give up some-thing pleasurable, such as being able to eat whatever you want when-ever you like, or sitting around watching TV rather than exercising, to get something more pleasurable: being thin? In many cases, the mas-ters seem to do a mental about-face and go from being passive vic-tims of their weight problems to being in control. Jeff B. describes "an audible click" that occurred in his head when he knew he was ready to lose weight permanently.

Like Kay, you can begin the process by looking within and asking yourself what kind of person you might be if you licked your weight problem. What is your weight keeping you from doing? How do you perceive yourself when you are heavy, and how does that conflict with what you'd like to be and do? How would you feel if you lost weight?

Now for the drawbacks. Ask yourself what price you would have to pay—in terms of money, time, pleasure, responses of others—to lose the weight and keep it off. Joanne F. (profiled in Chapter Five), who has kept 80 pounds at bay for 8 years, went so far as to commit the pros of losing weight to paper.

Your list might look something like this:

| PROS of Losing Weight | CONS of Losing Weight |
|---|---|
| I'll have more confidence. | I'll have to give up some foods I like. |
| I can wear more stylish clothes. | I don't like low-fat foods. |
| My spouse will be more attracted to me. | I'll have to spend money on new clothes. |
| My body will be healthier. | I'll have to spend money on a weight-loss program. |
| I'll be able to walk without getting out of breath. | I'll have to take time to plan meals. |
| I'll have more energy. | I hate to exercise. |
| People will stop staring at me because of my weight. | I'll have to learn some new recipes. |
| I'll be able to buy normal-size clothing. | My family may get angry because I won't buy certain foods. |
| I'll be able to do more with my children. | |
| My blood pressure will be lower. | |

As you tackle your weight problem, keep your list of "pros" handy at all times, add to it and refer to it frequently. This can help you reach the point at which changing your eating habits will be worth it— eventually, you'll want to be thinner more than you'll want to continue to engage in the behaviors that keep you from losing weight permanently. Dr. James Prochaska, Ph.D., coauthor of *Changing for Good*, believes that the reason so many people fail to change habits permanently is that they jump to action before they are truly ready— before they have fully accepted the fact that the long-term benefits of changing far outweigh any sacrifices.

## Want to Be Thin—But Not Too Thin

**M**ASTER CONNYE Z. SAYS IT BEST: "Being thinner—not thin— is the goal. Select a realistic weight for yourself." Connye is talking about what I call a "comfortable body weight"—one that you can maintain without undue suffering and one that causes no serious medical problems. And, for many masters, their comfortable body weight—the one they now maintain—is somewhat heavier than their "dream" weight, their original goal or what the charts "say" they should weigh. Connye states, "I got down to 116, and I was there for several years. But I have since gained 5 pounds. My weight fluctuates between 119 and 122, and that's pretty much where I stay."

## Try, Then Try Again

**I**F YOU HAVE FAILED MANY TIMES BEFORE and dread doing so again, it may help to know that, like Kay, most masters lost and regained many times before slimming down permanently. Stan J. (profiled in Chapter Two), who finally dropped more than 100 pounds, advises, "Try, then try again, again and again." He notes that even though he regained weight previously, his earlier experience helped him in his final try.

Although some reports have suggested that yo-yo dieting is harmful and makes it easier for you to gain weight in the future, it now appears you can lay to rest these concerns. A recent *Journal of the American Medical Association* review of dozens of studies on the effects of repeatedly gaining and losing weight (known as weight cycling) concludes: "There is no convincing evidence that weight cycling in humans has adverse effects on body composition, energy expenditure, risk factors for cardiovascular disease or the effectiveness of future efforts at weight loss." Most important, the report adds that there is no compelling reason to think yo-yo dieting is riskier than remaining obese. Because gaining, losing and gaining again can be psychologically painful, however, it may be better to wait until you are truly committed to making permanent lifestyle changes.

When she made her final weight-loss effort, Kay decided to focus on the future. She explains, "When I had thoughts like, 'You know you failed in the past,' I tried to push them out of my mind and replace them with positive images. I wanted to be the person that I knew was in there wanting to come out all those years."

# Take It One Day at a Time

ANOTHER WAY TO INCREASE YOUR BELIEF in your ability to change is, in the words of Kay, "Take it a day at a time. When I started, not only was I overweight, but I had little confidence in myself. So I decided to do it 5 pounds at a time. I didn't look at losing 75 to 80 pounds, because I figured that was going to set me up for failure."

Many other masters stress how wise it is to take things slow and steady. Patsy K., who is 99 pounds lighter than her all-time high, tells how it works: "I changed my eating habits over a long period. You can't change all of your bad habits at once. I still take one day at a time. When I fall, I pick myself up and start all over again. As long as I can accept the days I fail and put them behind me, then I will be able to maintain my goal."

# Never Forget Why You Lost the Weight

**W**HILE YOU'RE ACTIVELY LOSING WEIGHT, it's exciting to see the numbers on the scale drop and to witness other people's reactions as you dwindle away. But with time, the thinner you is no longer the "new" you, the compliments taper off and some people in your life don't even know you were once heavy.

When I asked the masters, "How do you stay motivated?" I got similar responses over and over. *The masters recall the pain of being heavy and never forget why they lost the weight.* Comments about their former lives as heavy people were among the most common responses:

◆ "I remember the pain, the rejection of being superfat." —Bob W. (246 pounds, 23 years)

◆ "Like the alcoholic who never wants to go back to alcohol, I NEVER want to go back. I hated that fat life." —Cindy P. (80 pounds, 12 years)

◆ "I will never go back to such pain. I deserve better. I want to keep my gorgeous clothes!" —Ann F. (220 pounds, 11 years)

◆ "I will always remember how I was, and I'll never be that again." —Terri M. (449 pounds, 3 years)

◆ "I remember the days of wearing a maxi pad every day of the month, because it kept my pant seam from digging into my butt. Being slim feels so good. I'll never let myself go back to being an overweight woman!" —Katie G. (30 pounds, 7 years)

To help keep herself going, Kay says, she reviews old photographs of herself. "In one photo, I am with my tiny Doberman puppy, and I'm kneeling down—I look like a sumo wrestler. I'm in a sleeveless tank top, and you should see my arms. I was fat!"

Likewise, Michael F. explains that he stays motivated to keep off his 137 pounds by looking at "before" pictures. He elaborates, "I remember what I went through to get to where I am and how much more I enjoy my present life."

Never forgetting why you lost the weight is not the same as dwelling on past failures. It is recalling the pain of being heavy in an effort to keep yourself from going back to your old food and exercise habits. I strongly suspect that one reason the masters feel compelled to recall the past is so that they don't become complacent. Kay admits, "I'm beating this thing, but I know that if I let my guard down, it could reverse itself." JoAnna L., who has kept off 130 pounds for 3 years, sums up: "I remember how I felt both physically and emotionally when I was 130 pounds heavier, and I don't want to feel that way again. I now live in the future, but I haven't completely forgotten the past."

# Celebrate the Benefits

A FTER THEY TELL YOU how they never forget the pain of being heavy, in the next breath, the masters invariably talk about how wonderful their lives are now. Kay says, "There are so many more fun things for me to do than eat. I like to go to the movies, go to the mall, do things with my grandchildren, go to the beach." In short, the masters look better, they feel better, they're healthier and they can do more things. And they have learned to celebrate the benefits.

◆ Whitney V. (72 pounds, 3 years): "I feel physically fit. I don't want to be fat again. I love buying clothes and bathing suits and fitting into airplane seats and bathrooms!"

◆ Katie G. (30 pounds, 7 years): "I zip up my jeans and notice my flat tummy! I tuck in my shirts. I go to stores and try on clothes and know I can choose an outfit because I like it—not because it does a fair job of hiding a protruding tummy."

◆ Maxine D. (39 pounds, 12 years): "My health is too improved to want to go back to old habits. After 22 years of pills, my doctor has taken me off all but one prescription drug. My blood pressure is normal. My cholesterol is good too."

◆ Eric Y. (27 pounds, 10 years): "How much more positive reinforcement does someone need than feeling better?"

The more I talk with the masters, the more I get the sense that losing weight permanently is one of the greatest accomplishments of their lives. It is the awareness of this accomplishment that underlies all their specific strategies and enables the masters to keep eating the way they do to stay thinner for life.

CHAPTER TWO

## Food Secret #2:

# Eat "Large"

OW HARD DO YOU HAVE TO WORK if you want to eat to stay
thin for life? Do you have to count calories and fat grams forever? Although some masters admit that they were obsessive at
first, with time, most seem to have been able to relax about food.
After they have at least several years of maintenance under their belts,
most do what *New York Times* health columnist Jane Brody so aptly
describes as "eating by concept" rather than "by number." Jane is
herself a master—she's lost 32 pounds and kept it off for 26 years.

Very few masters (6 out of 208, to be exact) said they count grams
of fat in food now that they're well into the maintenance stage. In fact,
a number of them stated that they really don't know exactly how much
fat they consume. Since most seem to eat "by concept," I decided to
look for the broad overriding principles that enable the masters to
stick to their commitment to a new food life.

*It all kept coming back to Stan J.'s words, "I figured out how to eat
large—and I do eat large."* He is referring to the essence of the masters'
new way of eating: They have learned how to get the most for their calories. They seek out foods that will fill them up but are not fattening.

## Stan J.'s Story

OW DOES A MAN who, for 50-some years, lived on rib-eye steaks,
French cuisine, ice cream, fried eggs and fettuccine Alfredo, arrive
at the point where he can say, "I eat low-fat and nonfat foods,
limit red meats, consume lots of broth-based soups and consciously

29

eat lots of vegetables and fruits"? How did this big-time meat-eater and, in his words, "lover of lush cuisine" finally drop 100-plus pounds and stay at his new weight for more than 5 years? For Stan, it took the shake-up of learning how seriously his health was in jeopardy.

His weight started to become a problem when he was in his mid-20s, after he got married. By the time he got divorced, at the age of 33, the scale had gradually climbed to 220, a hefty amount for a man who is just 5'7½". A marriage counselor suggested that he lose some weight, so on his own, he dropped 60 pounds, but he began to gain it back when he became involved in a new relationship. The relationship ended, but Stan's weight gain did not.

The turning point came in 1989, when he bumped into an old friend at a Christmas party. "I walked up to Bill to shake hands and wish him a happy holiday. But he didn't say, 'Happy holidays'; he didn't say, 'Hello.' He said, 'You need to lose weight. When you're ready to make a commitment, I will tell you the name of someone who can help you.' " Bill wouldn't give Stan the name until he had taken the weekend to think it over. He told Stan, "Call me on Monday, and when you're ready to make the commitment, I'll tell you who it is."

On Monday, Stan made the call. His friend referred him to the local Health Management Resources (HMR) weight-control program, which offers a medically supervised liquid "fasting" diet, as well as a comprehensive maintenance component. Although Stan had many physical problems, he had never associated them with being overweight—until he went to the orientation meeting.

For starters, he had sleep apnea (a condition that periodically interrupts breathing, causing the sleeper to awake) and a hiatal hernia (which causes acid reflux and heartburn). "I was sleeping in a vertical position. I couldn't walk a quarter of a mile without having my back hurt, and I'd have to sit down." Although he had stopped smoking three months earlier, he had "a cough that wouldn't quit." He remembers, "The meeting was in a lecture hall, way up high. I thought to myself, 'If I have to go to the bathroom and I get stuck in the middle with somebody just as large alongside of me, I'm dead.' I felt that if I got out of that chair, I might roll down the tier of seats."

Stan stayed on the liquid diet, taking weekly classes with the other participants for 18 weeks, until he got down to a weight of 175. After he had lost about 50 pounds, his cough went away, the pain in his back disappeared and he was able to sleep through the night. Today, he fluctuates between 180 and 190 pounds.

When the fast was over, Stan was taught how to reintroduce "real" foods gradually. For the next 18 months, he went to maintenance classes, learning about the importance of keeping food records, counting calories, weighing and measuring food and exercising. He was also told that it was critical to eat five servings of vegetables and/or fruits every day. "We figured out that to maintain my new weight, I could eat about 2,000 to 2,200 calories a day—more if I exercise a lot. Basically, I could eat anything I wanted, as long as I accounted for it and as long as I was sure to get in my vegetables and fruits."

Because Stan has a big appetite, he soon found himself taking advantage of his calorie book to come up with ways to get a large volume of food for his 2,000 or so calories so he could "eat large."

"If, instead of my customary rib-eye steak, I ate a skinless chicken breast or halibut steak, I discovered that I could eat twice as much food for the same calorie level. And if, instead of four or five slices of pizza with sausage, I ate two slices of my own vegetarian pizza with a big salad, I could get full on a lot less calories." Although the focus of his maintenance program was primarily on keeping track of *calories* in food, Stan found that he was automatically eating a low-fat diet, with about 20 percent of calories from fat.

To this day—five years after losing his weight—Stan still "eats large," going by two guiding principles he learned from his maintenance program: "First, all foods must be low-fat. Second, I eat lots of vegetables and fruits." But now, his habits require less thought. "The healthful choices have become instinctive." He does less weighing and measuring of foods because he is able to "project weights and volumes visually."

Stan eats three meals a day, and if he's hungry, he has a few snacks. Breakfast typically consists of a banana, half a bagel or a slice of dry whole-grain toast, a small apple and an ounce of cereal (such as Cheerios) topped with several ounces of fat-free yogurt. For lunch, he might have a broth-based soup—like chicken noodle or vegetable—along with a low-fat sandwich made with turkey breast or grilled vegetables. He often finishes the meal with a small fat-free or low-fat frozen yogurt cone. A typical dinner would consist of four ounces of baked or broiled chicken or seafood with herbs, several cups of vegetables and one to two cups of carbohydrate-rich foods, such as potato, pasta or rice. He snacks on fruits like apples or melon and sometimes makes himself a huge fruit salad that lasts for several days. "I don't need much rich, fancy or exotic food now," Stan says. "The simple pleasure of eating natural food in its basic form is great."

# Do Your Homework

L IKE STAN, most masters have to do their homework before they can relax and enjoy a new way of eating. Although many had a general sense of how they should eat before they lost the weight— for instance, they knew they should eat less fried food, avoid butter and eat more vegetables—they didn't know how to implement this knowledge as they ate three or more meals a day, 7 days a week, 365 days a year for a lifetime.

A number of masters indicated that they embarked on their new lives by making a concerted effort to learn which foods have fat in them and which don't and which foods are lowest in calories. Some took classes and some worked with registered dietitians, while others read books as well as newspaper and magazine articles. Many examined labels to learn more about food. (Masters who lose weight with a nondieting approach—by making an effort to eat healthfully, cut back on fat and exercise more—appear to have done most of their homework up front. Those who went the dieting route seemed to do much of it after they reached their goal weight.)

During the maintenance part of his program, Stan had to keep track of the fat in every item he ate for a month. At first, he stuck with foods that were easy to evaluate and simple to prepare. For instance, supper might be a baked potato, a cup or two of broccoli, three to four ounces of turkey and a slice of bread. With time, he began to introduce new and more complicated foods, but he remained fussy about their preparation—whether he was doing his own cooking or eating in a restaurant. He notes, "At first, I didn't feel comfortable about what I was doing or my ability to figure out foods. It didn't happen until I had gone through several books of record keeping."

# "Large" Lasts Longer

A FASCINATING RESEARCH ARTICLE in the *European Journal of Clinical Nutrition* makes it crystal-clear why Stan's concept of eating large works. In the first study of its kind, researchers from the University of Sydney, Australia, developed a sort of index of food satisfaction. Participants were asked to rate foods in six different categories— from fruits to bakery products—according to how full they felt after eating them.

Calorie for calorie, foods that were higher in fat were rated low for creating a sense of fullness. Conversely, foods that were low in fat— but high in fiber and water—were rated more filling. Why? Because the more-filling foods netted a much larger portion for a 240-calorie serving, *and* they took longer to eat. For instance, a 240-calorie portion of French fries was only about 3 ounces, while a portion of plain boiled potatoes was about 12 ounces; a serving of fatty Cheddar cheese was 2 ounces, while a serving of lean steamed fish was 11 ounces. Boiled potatoes, the most filling food, were ranked seven times more filling than croissants, the least filling food. In the snack category, popcorn was twice as filling as a Mars Bar or peanuts. Whole-grain versions of products, such as bread, pasta and cereal, were considered more filling than their more refined counterparts. And the effect of the more-filling foods lasted. Two hours after eating the more-filling foods—when the tasters were allowed to eat freely of assorted foods and drinks—they tended to eat less.

The study also showed that the protein content of foods influenced how filling they were. The authors note, "Protein-rich foods . . . have consistently been found to produce stronger and more sustained feelings of fullness and decrease food intake later than foods high in fat or sucrose [sugar]." The message is that your meals are likely to stay with you longer if you include a small portion of a low-fat protein food, such as fish, chicken or reduced-fat cheese. (For a comparison of two menus—one filling and low-fat, the other high-fat—see page 39.)

# How to "Eat Large"

In describing their eating habits, the masters mentioned four basic strategies again and again.

## Strategy #1

**Choose low-fat over high-fat.** The guiding principle for the vast majority of masters is low-fat eating. When asked, "Do you eat a low-fat diet now?" 9 out of 10 said "Yes." Moreover, comments about low-fat eating dominated the masters' general responses about how they eat. Most masters told me they consume in the neighborhood of 20 to 30 percent of their calories from fat. (To get an idea of how many grams you can have on varying calorie levels, see the opposite page.)

The masters have learned that when you cut back on fat, you get to eat a greater volume of food for any given calorie level. As Jennifer P. sums up, "With lower-fat foods, you can be full or satisfied most of the time."

Simply stated, the masters have discovered that fat begets fat. Patsy B., who's kept off 104 pounds for 4 years, probably doesn't know how close she is to the biochemical truth when she explains, "I always think that the fat I put in my mouth will end up on my body, and it takes way too long to get it out of my system. It's not worth eating." Similarly, Joanna M., a 12-year master with a 51-pound loss, advises, "When you're tempted to eat something high-fat, think about a fat place on your body that you wish were thinner and remember how easily the body stores fat because it's already in the right form."

# HOW MUCH FAT FOR YOUR CALORIES?

**M**OST MASTERS CONSUME in the neighborhood of 20 to 30 percent of their calories from fat. The following chart shows how many grams of fat you can consume on varying calorie levels.

| IF YOU EAT THIS MANY CALORIES | YOU CAN HAVE THIS MUCH FAT IN GRAMS for 20% calories from fat | for 30% calories from fat |
|---|---|---|
| 1,200 | 27 g | 40 g |
| 1,300 | 29 g | 43 g |
| 1,400 | 31 g | 47 g |
| 1,500 | 33 g | 50 g |
| 1,600 | 36 g | 53 g |
| 1,700 | 38 g | 57 g |
| 1,800 | 40 g | 60 g |
| 1,900 | 42 g | 63 g |
| 2,000 | 44 g | 67 g |
| 2,100 | 47 g | 70 g |
| 2,200 | 49 g | 73 g |
| 2,300 | 51 g | 77 g |
| 2,400 | 53 g | 80 g |

There are two main reasons why choosing low-fat over high-fat works:

**1. Fat is the most fattening nutrient.** With its 9 calories per gram, fat has more than double the calories of the other calorie-yielding nutrients, carbohydrate and protein, each of which provides 4 calories per gram. (A gram is about one-thirtieth of an ounce.) Another way to think of it is that an ounce of fat has approximately 270 calories, while an ounce of either pure protein or carbohydrate has just 120 calories. Thus your intake of calories can jump quite markedly when you consume even small amounts of high-fat items.

Indeed, studies suggest that when people are allowed to eat freely of high-fat foods, they consume significantly more calories than when they're allowed to eat all they want of low-fat foods. In one Cornell University experiment in which participants were offered diets of three different fat levels and told they could eat as much as they liked, they consumed an average of about 500 calories more per day on the highest-fat diet than on the lowest. In short, when the diet is rich in fat, people tend to consume more calories than they need.

**2. The body is efficient at storing food fat as body fat.** While eating too much of *any* of the calorie-yielding nutrients can make you gain weight, excess fat calories are more readily converted to body fat than are excess carbohydrate or protein calories. The reason is that the body actually burns some calories as it processes proteins, carbohydrates and fats, because it takes some effort to digest and metabolize them. It takes less effort and thus burns fewer calories to process fat than the other two nutrients. According to obesity researcher James O. Hill, Ph.D., of the University of Colorado Health Sciences Center, 90 percent of excess fat calories are converted to body fat, while only 70 percent of excess carbohydrate calories are shifted to body fat.

This does not mean you can eat all you want of low-fat foods and still lose weight: too many calories—whether low-fat or not—can still add up. (For more on the importance of watching calories, see Chapter Three.)

In eating low-fat, the masters do the obvious—choose baked and broiled foods over fried versions, choose nonfat and low-fat dairy products over whole-milk products and choose low-fat baked goods like bread and bagels over breakfast pastries and rich desserts. But probably the most significant way they cut fat is to, in the words of Mabel H., "refrain from using visible fats—butter, margarine, salad dressings, cream." Mabel is referring to the most concentrated fat culprits, the "added" fats, which also include oil, shortening, lard and mayonnaise. (Because of their high-fat content, regular cream cheese, sour cream, bacon and avocados are considered added fats too.) When asked how often they use butter and regular margarine, more than 100 masters answered "Never," "Almost never" or "Once or twice a month." Another 40 masters use butter or margarine no more than four times a week. Joanna M. sees it this way, "Forgoing butter means you can have an entire extra roll with the calories you saved." As Lynda C. (41 pounds, 6 years) states, "I played the numbers game for years. Now, fat grams are my gauge. But I don't count them, and I never know what you're supposed to get each day. All I know is, I prefer not to slap a pat of butter on my potato, and I eat no fried foods or cream sauces."

The masters motivate themselves to avoid fatty foods in different ways. Ann Q. uses imagery to deter herself: "A high-fat-content item reminds me of a layer of lard sitting on top of a food item. Or I think 'heart attack on a plate' . . . that gets *my* attention."

A number of masters seem to have reached the point where they actually have an aversion to fatty foods, as Debbie T. illustrates, "I can't stand greasy fried foods—yuck!" Lynda C. says, "I don't know how I changed my palate, but the plainer, the better. If I throw pork chops or chicken breasts in the oven, it's with a lemon wedge, some parsley and some onions. I absolutely prefer to eat this way."

**Take it slow.** There is no question that when you're accustomed to higher-fat foods, a low-fat way of eating takes some getting used to. So as Vicki B. (61 pounds, 10 years) puts it, "Be patient with your taste buds. It takes a little while to adjust." Debbie T., who's kept off 62 pounds for more than 6 years, offers this advice for changing your food habits gradually: "To begin a low-fat diet, start changing things you eat little by little. Instead of eating a doughnut for breakfast, eat a bagel. Instead of spaghetti with cream sauce, try a tomato-based sauce. Little by little, make your changes. It takes some time."

The good news is that research evidence suggests that the desire for fatty foods is an acquired or learned taste rather than something we're born with. Thus you can "unlearn" a desire for fat-laden foods.

Milk is a great example of how this works. Most baby boomers grew up drinking whole milk and found it difficult to switch to skim. Now, many actually prefer skim.

Each time you're about to add a spoonful of mayonnaise, a pat of margarine or a ladle of salad dressing, ask yourself, "Could I enjoy this with half the fat or maybe even no fat?" Many people find they can get used to certain foods, such as warm bagels and bread, without any extra fat.

The masters are big users of the numerous reduced-fat and fat-free products on the market, and they advise experimenting. In the words of Julie R., "Don't let one bad-tasting low-fat product be a final decision for all low-fat products." Don't feel you have to abandon all regular fats—just use them sparingly. Stan J. uses olive oil in small amounts, while Cathy B. uses butter, but she adds, "Never more than one tablespoon per day."

Jennifer P. recommends, "Keep the flavor, lose the fat." She uses low-fat or fat-free margarine and mayonnaise, as well as such low-fat or nonfat additions as barbecue sauce, catsup and spices. Similarly, Patsy B. uses lots of fat-free dressings on salads, potatoes and pasta. To jazz up bagels, she spreads on jelly, jam, apple butter or honey—all of which are fat-free. Now 60 pounds lighter for 8 years, Chuck B. adds, "People need to understand that low-fat doesn't mean boring. Matter of fact, you'll find it tastes *better*."

> *Following are two sample meals consisting of the same number of calories. Menu #1 contains more than three times the fat of Menu #2. Think about how much fuller you'd feel on the low-fat plan, which affords you about three times as much food—40 ounces versus 14 ounces.*

# How "Eating Large" Works

| Menu #1 | Amount | Calories | Fat (grams) |
|---|---|---|---|
| Fried Chicken | 4 ounces | 305 | 17 |
| French Fries | 10-12 (2 ounces) | 179 | 9 |
| Coleslaw | ½ cup | 89 | 7 |
| Biscuit | one | 127 | 6 |
| Cheesecake | ½ cake | 295 | 21 |
| with Strawberry | | | |
| Topping | 2 tablespoons | 108 | 0 |
| | | | |
| **Totals:** | **14 ounces** | **1,103** | **60** |

| Menu #2 | Amount | Calories | Fat (grams) |
|---|---|---|---|
| Skinless Roast | | | |
| Chicken Breast | 4 ounces | 187 | 4 |
| Large Baked Potato | 6½ ounces | 201 | 0 |
| with Fat-Free | | | |
| Sour Cream | 3 tablespoons | 47 | 0 |
| Steamed Peas | | | |
| and Carrots | 1 cup | 77 | 1 |
| Tossed Green Salad | 2 cups | 50 | 1 |
| with Fat-Free | | | |
| Salad Dressing | 3 tablespoons | 75 | 0 |
| Dinner Rolls | 2 | 170 | 4 |
| Margarine | 1 teaspoon | 34 | 4 |
| Angel Food Cake | ⅒ cake | 183 | 1 |
| with Sliced Fresh | | | |
| Strawberries | 1 cup | 50 | 1 |
| and Lite Whipped | | | |
| Topping | 3 tablespoons | 30 | 2 |
| | | | |
| **Totals:** | **40 ounces** | **1,104** | **18** |

# Strategy #2

**Veg out.** One of Stan's most important principles for eating large is, "I eat as many vegetables as I can." The night before I interviewed him, his dinner consisted of: 4 ounces of Cajun broiled halibut, 3 cups of steamed broccoli, 1 cup of steamed baby carrots and a salad consisting of 6 cups of torn lettuce, a little pineapple, ⅓ ounce pine nuts, nonfat raspberry-vinaigrette dressing and a sprinkling of Parmesan cheese. Stan also goes out of his way to eat fruit at least two or three times a day. He's not alone: Most of the masters eat vegetables at least two or three times a day, and many enjoy fruits that frequently. Vegetables and fruits are virtually fat-free, and they're high in fiber and volume for the number of calories they contain. In Ann F.'s words, "Fruits and salads help fill you up. I eat large quantities of vegetables and ample fruits but use moderation in other foods." Similarly, Emil R. uses vegetables to help him limit portions of other foods. "I take average portions of foods and enjoy. If I still feel hungry after giving myself time to feel full, I take seconds of veggies. *They* didn't get me up to 335 pounds!" This method has helped him keep his weight at 220 for 9 years. (He's 6'4½".)

The take-home message from the masters seems to be that you should try to eat *at least* five servings of vegetables and fruits a day. Most of them likely eat far more than this, as does Jane Brody: "My portions of vegetables are large—double or triple the half-cup standard." (For portion sizes of fruits and vegetables, see page 56.) Salads seem to factor into masters' meal planning in a big way—as you'll see in Part II "Meals from the Masters,"—probably because lettuce is so filling and almost calorie-free. But beware the dressing (a small ladleful can easily scoop up several hundred calories) as well as other higher-fat goodies that often accompany salads—like croutons, cheese and sunflower seeds—especially at salad bars. It has been reported that students whose food came from a cafeteria salad bar actually ate more calories and fat than did students who got all their food from the "hot line."

# 13 WAYS TO EAT MORE FRUITS AND VEGETABLES

**1. Try at least one new vegetable or fruit each week.** To enliven meals, switch from the old, familiar green beans, apples and bananas to okra, winter squash, papaya and kiwi.

**2. Eat more "meal" salads.** Use a large salad as the base, but throw in meat "condiments"—several ounces of cooked chicken, turkey, tuna or some low-fat cheese and/or legumes. Add warm bread, and you've got a complete meal.

**3. Put fruit in your vegetables.** Add sliced or chopped apples, pears, grapes, melon, kiwi and orange sections to tossed, spinach and cabbage salads. (See Fruits and Greens in Raspberry Vinaigrette, page 283.) You can even combine cooked vegetables with fruit—for instance, Sweet Potato Puff (page 294) contains bananas.

**4. Take advantage of ready-made bag salads.** These are great when you're in a rush or feeling tired. Look for fresh ingredients, and add a low-fat or fat-free dressing. Experiment with some of the darker greens, like Romaine and leaf lettuce—they're tastier and more nutritious.

**5. Have at least one fruit serving with each meal.** It's easy. For instance, have a banana or strawberries on cereal, a piece of fresh fruit with your lunch and/or as a snack and a fruit serving with dinner. (If you don't feel like cooking a vegetable or making a salad, slice up some cantaloupe or honeydew melon.)

**6. If you're in the dessert habit, try substituting fruit,** served in a creative way, in place of at least three desserts a week. For instance, try an apple baked with some cinnamon and a few raisins, a banana with a small amount of reduced-fat peanut butter, a bowl of fresh, juicy mixed berries, or a big serving of fruit on top of a small serving of frozen yogurt or angel food cake. (To save on unwanted calories, avoid fruit canned or frozen in heavy syrup or with added sugar.)

**7. Experiment with nonfat flavorings.** Sprinkle nutmeg and lemon juice on spinach or broccoli, dill weed and Dijon-style mustard on green beans or carrots, and basil on tomatoes.

**8. Mix your vegetables.** For example, combine corn and beans, zucchini and onions, red potato and carrot slivers, eggplant and tomatoes, cucumbers and onions. Frozen mixtures without sauce are fine too.

**9. Eat more vegetable-rich main dishes.** For instance, try Shrimp and Pepper Mexicana (page 232) or Vegetable Tofu Stir-Fry (page 262).

**10. Combine vegetables with tasty broths and juices.** Green beans cooked in chicken broth, summer squash in tomato juice, and carrots or beets in fruit juice are flavorful and need no added fat.

**11. Have at least one vegetable at lunchtime.** Take along ready-to-eat carrots, cucumbers and celery with fat-free salad dressing. If there's a refrigerator at work, keep these items on hand.

**12. Be creative with low-fat potato toppings.** Try salsa, nonfat cheese, nonfat sour cream with chives, fat-free butter spray and a few bacon bits, fat-free salad dressings, low-fat chili or low-fat cottage cheese with dill weed.

**13. Try roasting or grilling vegetables.** Roasted vegetables taste heartier and more flavorful than steamed or boiled ones, and they are easy to prepare. Coat chunks of peppers, zucchini, summer squash, onions, eggplant or firm tomatoes with a light coating of vegetable spray or marinate them in a low-fat dressing, and grill or bake at 400 degrees F for about 15 minutes, turning occasionally.

# Strategy #3

**Go for grains.** Like many masters, Stan also eats large by regularly eating pasta and rice, as well as whole-grain breads and cereals—all of which are virtually fat-free. A quick glance at the masters' meal plans reveals that a number of them are heavy pasta consumers. In fact, Kay D. eats pasta just about every day. "When I eat more pasta and vegetables for my main meal, they keep me full for the rest of the afternoon." (One of her tricks for eating large is to cook pasta for a long time so it plumps with water and takes on more volume.)

More than one-third of the masters indicated that they eat pasta or rice at least three or four times a week, and about 40 percent of them eat cold or hot cereal that often; nearly half of the masters noted that they have bread at least two or three times a day. Jennifer P. states, "Finding out that I could eat more carbohydrates has really helped me maintain." Paul A. adds that compared with when he was heavy, "I have increased my intake of high-starch foods, such as crisp breads and bagels."

Lately, the old-fashioned notion that bread, pasta, rice and the like are fattening has been receiving renewed attention in the media, usually in connection with the supposed benefits of a high-protein diet. However, the masters' eating habits are just the opposite. And their habits are supported by most professionals. As the *Harvard Health Letter* states, "Pasta is not poison . . . pasta and other carbohydrate-rich foods will not make people fat—unless they eat too much of them." (See portion sizes of grain foods, page 56, and "A Low-Fat Portion Is Still a Portion," page 59.)

To boost your fiber intake, it's wise to take Stan's lead in selecting whole-grain versions of bread and cereal products whenever possible. Good bets for fiber are breads with whole wheat flour listed as the first ingredient, whole wheat pasta, brown rice, barley, bulgur, oat bran, oatmeal and whole-grain cereals (compare labels for fiber content). Fiber-rich foods may help with weight control because they tend to take longer to eat, and fiber can slow down the rate at which the stomach empties. Some studies have shown that when compared with low-fiber foods, high-fiber foods eaten at breakfast or at lunch significantly reduce the amount consumed at the next meal.

# Strategy #4

**Lighten up on meats.** The masters not only eat *less* meat but they generally favor light-colored "meats"—namely, poultry and seafood, which also tend to be "light" in fat and calories. Stan's habits are typical. He says, "I know that in general, fish has the least fat, then chicken, then red meat. So I limit consumption of red meats and follow a modified vegetarian diet that includes fish and chicken."

Like Stan, scores of masters reported that they eat little or no red meat. Of the 208 masters surveyed, about 130 indicated that they eat meat once or twice a week at the most. When I asked them open-endedly how they would describe their current eating habits, comments about eating less meat were the second most prevalent responses, after comments about eating less fat.

Knowing that from a nutritional perspective there is no reason to exclude lean meats, I ask Stan why he doesn't just eat the leaner cuts. He replies, "Red meat brings back the memory of how I used to eat. I just didn't feel right when I had it."

When I ask Kay D. why she decided to become a vegetarian, she explains, "I didn't intentionally set out this way. But after a year or two, I gradually lost my taste for meat and started eating more pasta and vegetables." In place of meats, many masters have legumes, such as chick-peas, kidney beans, navy beans, pinto beans and lentils. They seem to eat legumes more often than does the average American— nearly 40 percent have them at least once or twice a week.

While a number of masters don't eliminate red meat entirely, they do make an effort to limit portion sizes and to "stretch" it. (For portion sizes of meats, poultry and fish, see page 57.) Linda M. says, "I use meat as a condiment." Molly A. is on the same wavelength: "I use small amounts of meat or chicken for flavor and interest." Karen S. agrees, "Think of meat as an 'ingredient,' as in stir-fries, Mexican and pasta dishes." If meat is served by itself, Karen recommends having it with plenty of other low-fat foods—for example, with bread, potato, salad and a vegetable. She adds, "If you have seconds at a meal, have the nonprotein portions."

# Building a New "Library of Food"

I N LEARNING HOW TO EAT LARGE, the masters seem to have reached a point where they prefer the way they are now eating to their old ways. Carole B., who's kept off 71 pounds, affirms, "You make a lifelong change and feel better for it." Stan says, "Throw out your old concepts about what should and shouldn't taste good. The other day, I tossed together a big salad of fresh spinach, crumbled pretzels, fat-free poppy-seed dressing and warm chunks of baked potato—it was delicious. Eating large has led me to a whole new library of food. I can stay alive longer and eat more."

## CHAPTER THREE

## Food Secret #3:

# Fix Your Full Button

WOULDN'T IT BE NICE if we could all simply eat when we're hungry and stop when we're full? The truth is, it just doesn't seem to work this way for most masters. As Don Mauer puts it, "My full button *is* broken, not *was* broken. For me, 'full' is what most people feel after Thanksgiving dinner. When it's painful, I am full." Even 5 years into maintenance, Don still has a tendency to eat beyond the point of being full.

You may be wondering whether "eating large" will take care of this—if you fill up on low-fat foods, like vegetables and pasta, won't you be okay? Not totally, because the concept of getting the most for your calories works only to a point. Things can still get out of hand, and you may wind up eating too many calories.

Thus even though the masters tend to eat large, they still keep a lid on the amount of food eaten at any one sitting, as they made clear when they answered my question, "How do you know when to stop eating?" *The vast majority responded that they take important steps to place limits on the amount of food they eat.*

## Don Mauer's Story

IT'S BEEN ABOUT FOUR YEARS NOW since Don Mauer came my way from the *Chicago Sun-Times* after I sent its food editor an announcement of my search for people who had lost weight and kept it off. The prominent newspaper had just profiled Don in a feature article about his remarkable weight loss of 100-plus pounds *and* his talent for developing "high-taste, low-fat" recipes. Don is one of a number of masters who have turned their weight-loss success into a vocation; he now writes a newspaper column, demonstrates low-fat cooking on television, teaches cooking classes and has just published his first cookbook, *Lean and Lovin' It* (Chapters Publishing, 1996).

Up until he was 10 years old, Don says, "I had bony knees and little skinny wrists; I have home movies to prove it." At that time, however, he started to get fat and stayed that way for four decades. Don vividly recalls when, as a third grader, it was his turn to tell the class about his Thanksgiving holiday: "I was enormously proud that I had eaten three helpings. That may have been the beginning of eating too much. It's when I discovered how good lots of food made me feel." By the time he was 15, Don weighed 207 pounds. (He is 5' 8½".)

In his 20s, Don remained in the low 200s, which is what he weighed when he got married at the age of 24. As Don worked his way up to more than 300 pounds, his morning "breakfast" would consist of a cigarette and a cup of coffee. Then, after going all day without eating, he'd come home and start cooking. He recalls, "I used to keep a bottle of Hershey's syrup on the refrigerator door so I could squirt a 'shot' of chocolate in my mouth as I was cooking. I would leave my butter sitting out so it would get soft. Then, while I was making dinner, I'd take saltines and scrape them down through the butter. I'd knock off half a stick of butter on saltines before we even sat down to eat."

His subsequent dinner might consist of a 12-ounce prime T-bone steak (topped with a pat of butter), vegetables with butter and bread with butter. Later, Don would reach for one of the 10 to 15 different flavors of Häagen Dazs ice cream he kept in his freezer, right next to his chocolate-covered graham crackers. He notes, "I would eat until I fell asleep in front of the television." Don also says that he went on food binges three to four times a week. "Over a two-to-three-hour period, I could consume a pound of M&M's or a pound or more of peanuts."

All the butter, premium ice cream and binge eating pushed Don's weight to over 300 pounds and skyrocketed his cholesterol to 240.

(A healthy cholesterol reading is under 200.) Finally, in January 1990, a holiday photograph of himself "tripped the switch," in Don's words, and prompted a visit to the medically supervised Optifast program at his local hospital. He stayed on a liquid diet for 12 weeks and lost 70 pounds. For the next six weeks, he gradually added back regular foods. Then he struck out on his own course of low-fat eating, consuming several meals a day and keeping his fat intake to less than 20 percent of his total calories.

He says, "When I discovered low-fat foods, it was almost like a miracle: I could get filled up on lower-calorie foods. For example, I reached full sooner, with fewer calories, on French bread than I did on peanuts and raisins. For a while, it didn't matter that my full button was broken, because I could eat a lot and still lose weight. I saw this as magical. And it was, for a while." Between the low-fat eating and brisk walking for 45 minutes several times a week, Don kept dropping 2 to 3 pounds a week, until he got down to his current maintenance weight range of 195 to 200; his cholesterol dropped to 158.

His weight stayed down for about three years, when he found out the hard way that low-fat eating isn't enough. He recounts, "I had just moved to North Carolina, and my food scale was in storage. It was a hot summer, and I started eating huge portions of cold homemade low-fat rice salad and pasta salad. I had also discovered a wonderful locally made sauerkraut-rye bread, which I was eating without butter with abandon. I thought I was safe; my food was about as low in fat as you can get—just 10 percent of my calories were coming from fat. But my jeans had gotten so tight that they hurt—I had to unbuckle them when I sat down to work. That's when I realized that calories count and low-fat isn't so magical after all."

Don has come to terms with the fact he has to watch *portion sizes* of foods—including low-fat foods. He still eats large, which helps to a point. But he is much more careful about portions, which he can pretty much assess by eye. In an effort to get away from the "compulsiveness" about what he ate in the first few years of maintenance, Don purposely avoids weighing, measuring and writing down *every* item he eats. But he still routinely uses his food scale to weigh and measure certain foods, such as meats and cereal. He notes, "The scale helps when you get sloppy." And when he finds himself on the up-side of his 195-to-200-pound weight range, he goes back to writing down everything he eats.

Don also plans his meals a week in advance, stocking up on health-ful foods so they're always on hand. To control his between-meal hunger, Don has recently been experimenting with eating more lean protein foods, like tuna and skinless chicken breast. He notes, "I found that when I was eating all-vegetable meals, I was starving an hour or two later."

When he starts to gain, he also avoids eating in front of the TV. "I go back to the dining room table and eat without extra stimuli so I can pay attention to what is on my plate and how much I put in my mouth. It also helps because I have someone across from me—my wife—watching how much I eat."

# Is Your Full Button Broken?

A s DON MAKES SO PAINFULLY CLEAR, eating large does not give you carte blanche to eat limitless portions. *You still have to get a grip on the amount of food that you eat at any one sitting.* Yes, there are some masters (about 1 out of 5) who seem to be able to stop eat-ing when they are full; they say they let their level of fullness be the determinant of how much they eat. These masters have developed a sensitivity to their body's physiological hunger cues so they know when to stop. Hazel U.'s policy is, "I try to stop *before* I start feeling full. I try to remember how miserable I'll feel if I overeat." And Jen-nifer B. has learned, "For the most part, it is okay to stop eating when I feel satisfied, not *stuffed*. I know I will eat again!" Bob W. adds, "I've learned to listen to my body. I ask myself, 'Am I really hungry?' " He stops eating when "just satisfied; I remember it's *not* my last meal." JoAnna L. says she has become more sensitive to her body's signals: "In the old days, even when I was learning to eat healthy, I would not have stopped until my plate was clean. I can now hear that inner voice telling me when I've had enough. It was a long time coming, but after tuning in to your own body, it really does happen."

But most masters cannot rely solely on their internal sense of satisfaction to tell them how much to consume. Linda W. explains one reason many people have difficulty: "I was taught as a child not to waste food, and cleaning my plate was a MUST. It was and still is hard to break that habit and to push away from the table when I haven't cleaned my plate."

*In an effort to break the habit of plate cleaning and to teach themselves not to eat beyond the point of being full, 1 out of 4 masters makes an effort to leave some food on his or her plate after each meal.* Molly A. offers an interesting technique for doing this: "Visualize what remains on your plate as (1) on your hips or (2) in the garbage can. Either the hips or the garbage can is going to get it. It really works." Once 227 pounds, she now weighs 143.

# Plan Ahead

WHEN I ASKED THE MASTERS, "What determines how much you eat at any one meal or snack? What determines when you stop eating?" their most common responses had to do with *planning ahead.* Not only do the masters plan *the general content of day-to-day meals* ahead of time—sometimes up to a week in advance—but *before they start eating, they decide how much they will serve themselves.* Kay D. remarks, "The important thing is that you're not caught off guard so that in a weak moment you can justify why you're going to eat something. I try to know ahead of time what kind of situation I'm getting into." She even goes so far as to call airlines ahead when she travels, to make sure she gets a low-fat meal. She also anticipates holidays and social events involving food.

**Planning day-to-day meals in advance** is a preventive step against impulse eating. Don Mauer plots out his suppers a week ahead. He explains how it works: "We have a fixed menu six out of seven nights. Two nights, we have pita pizza—pita bread with low-fat spaghetti sauce, low-fat mozzarella cheese, onions, sweet red pepper and a few sliced olives. We might have that with a cabbage slaw. One night, we have homemade soup with bread and a salad. Then we have a fish night—maybe salmon with oven-roasted potatoes and peas. We always have a vegetarian night—for example, baked potatoes with chives and freshly ground pepper, a large tossed salad with fat-free dressing and broccoli. Qn meat night, we might have lean hamburger or pork. The seventh night is 'wild-card night'—we'll try something new from a low-fat cookbook or magazine. If we love the new recipe a lot, it may become more of a mainstay."

Other masters plan their meals the night before. Lynda C. manages to think a day ahead, even with a baby, a three-quarter-time job and a husband who is frequently out at night (*and* who can eat whatever he wants). "At night, after the baby is asleep and I've eaten," she says, "I make lunch to take to work and will take something out to thaw for the next night's supper." Lynda has been a master for more than 6 years, down 41 pounds from her all-time high and just 4 pounds shy of her prepregnancy weight.

Although they plan their meals in advance, the masters allow for some give-and-take and realize that even the best-laid plans fail at times. As Lynda M. explains, "I try to plan my meals ahead, but if I exceed my planned intake, I cut back at the next meal."

**Stocking up.** You can't eat healthful foods if you don't have them around. So the masters make sure they've got the "right" stuff on hand, often by purchasing certain stock items each week at the grocery store. Don Mauer keeps on hand foods like pita bread, fresh and frozen vegetables, reduced-fat mozzarella cheese, pasta, low-fat spaghetti sauce and an assortment of cereal.

Likewise, Kay D. purchases the same foods weekly and says, "My husband can shop for me now, and he doesn't even have to ask what to get. My list includes Healthy Choice fat-free cheese, skim milk, Fiber One cereal, Mueller's macaroni, Hunt's unsalted whole canned tomatoes, bananas and other fruits. And I buy Texas Pete hot sauce by the gallon!"

**Planning how much to serve yourself.** *The masters go out of their way to limit portion sizes by serving themselves finite amounts.* As Jane Brody puts it, "Because I don't know when to stop eating, I must decide in advance how much I'm going to have. If I sit down with a box of graham crackers, I could eat a whole packet. Likewise, with a pint of frozen yogurt. So I set an amount ahead of time: two crackers, one bar of frozen yogurt." Like Jane Brody, many other masters have a tendency to eat whatever is put in front of them—even if it means eating beyond being full. Don Mauer, who to this day claims, "A portion of frozen yogurt for me can easily be a whole half-gallon container," says he limits the amount he eats as follows, "I don't overserve myself—then there's no temptation to fill up." Diane J. says, "I try never to eat more food at a time than the size of my fist." Lynda C. notes, "There are specific portions for each meal and type of food I eat. I try to stay within these boundaries. I fill my plate with portions that are healthy and try not to go for seconds." In fact, many masters make it a rule to avoid having second helpings.

Another technique that helps limit amounts eaten at any one sitting is to buy foods in preportioned amounts, especially if they're tempting foods. Connye Z. says, "I have trouble controlling my portions of ice cream, so I eat Weight Watchers desserts every night. There are two in a package. I love them, but I've never eaten them both because they're premeasured. If I get ice cream, however, I can scoop out as much as I want."

Other masters find it helps to use small-sized dishes or to use the same dish so they always know they're getting the same amount. Patsy K. states, "I use a small plate, a small bowl and a small cup. I have always cleaned my plate, so if I use a small one, I start out with less food."

It's not just heavy and formerly heavy people who have a tendency to overeat when they are served large helpings: For many of us, the more we see, the more we eat. In a recent study at the U.S. Army Research Center at Natick, Massachusetts, when normal-weight men were given three different-sized portions of macaroni and cheese (in random order), they ate significantly more as portions grew. On average, they consumed five ounces more when given the largest portion than they did when offered the smallest. (Five ounces of regular macaroni and cheese has about 200 calories and 10 grams of fat.)

Nancy K. goes by set portion sizes for most foods but fills any hunger void with low-fat, low-calorie items. She rarely allows herself seconds on "anything other than fruit and veggies." Similarly, Debbie T. states, "I know what a serving is supposed to be, and that is what I give myself. If I'm still hungry, I eat more fruits, vegetables or sometimes carbohydrates."

# The Pause That Finishes

SOME MASTERS LIMIT THE AMOUNT THEY EAT by finalizing their meals in a symbolic way. Joanna M. not only "plans the portion ahead of time" but finishes a meal with "a refreshing cold drink, hot coffee or tea or a mint—to get the taste of the food out of my mouth." Jennie C. says, "I usually put what I consider a balanced meal on the plate and rarely eat seconds. At the end of the meal, I brush my teeth and get that 'finished-with-food' feeling."

Finally, many masters—in fact, nearly half of them—find that if they make a conscious effort to slow down their rate of eating, it helps them limit the amount they eat at meals. "I eat slower and let my stomach fullness tell me when to stop," states Julie R., who's kept off 53 pounds for more than 10 years.

Some masters intentionally build a delay into their eating to slow themselves down. Bonnie R. explains her technique: "I put small portions on my plate and stop eating when my plate is empty. Since it takes 20 minutes for all the food to enter the stomach and fill it, I wait. If I'm still hungry, I may or may not eat more." Judy F. adds, "I pay attention to how I feel by trying not to eat fast and waiting 20 minutes before deciding whether or not I need more."

# Learn What a Portion Is

P ART AND PARCEL OF DECIDING HOW MUCH you are going to have is not kidding yourself about what a reasonable amount of food is. In other words, as Molly A. (84 pounds, 12 years) puts it, "I learned what a 'regular' portion is. Fat people don't know." In fact, many people tend to underestimate the amount of food they eat.

Some research suggests that obese individuals are particularly likely to report eating less food than they've actually had. Two recent studies of overweight people conducted at St. Luke's-Roosevelt Hospital in New York City found that although they reported eating less than 1,200 calories, most were, in fact, eating more than 2,000 calories.

Health Management Resources, a Boston-based weight-control program, offers some striking examples of how misjudging portion sizes can easily lead to weight gain:

◆ If you underestimate a bran muffin to weigh 1½ ounces instead of 3 ounces, the difference in calories is twofold: 150 versus 300.

◆ Figuring a 12-ounce steak to weigh 6 ounces (not an uncommon kind of mistake) leads to a 600-calorie underestimate.

These two errors alone add up to 750 calories or about half of the daily calorie requirement—at maintenance, *not* while dieting—for some women!

Be aware, too, that calorie books can be misleading. One of mine, for instance, lists a single bagel at 163 calories for 2 ounces. But the bagels from our local bagel shop actually weigh about 4 ounces and thus would have twice as many calories.

# Sizing Up Portions

J UDGING PORTION SIZES JUST BY LOOKING takes a lot of practice. To figure out how much to serve yourself, Catherine C. offers a tip that has worked for many masters: "Measure food until it is in your brain." Lynda C. agrees, "I absolutely pay attention to the amounts I eat. I used to weigh and measure, but now I gauge food by looking at it."

# ARE YOU KIDDING YOURSELF?

*Take the following quiz to see whether you're kidding yourself on portion control.*

1. An ounce and a half of hard cheese—equivalent to one serving from the dairy group—looks most like (a) one domino; (b) two dominoes; (c) three dominoes.

2. Half a cup of cooked pasta, considered a serving from the grain group, most easily fits into (a) an ice cream scoop (the kind with a release handle); (b) a ball the size of a medium grapefruit; (c) a cereal bowl.

3. Women are advised to have no more than one alcoholic drink a day. If that drink is wine, it should roughly fill (a) one coffee cup; (b) two-thirds of a coffee cup; (c) two coffee cups.

4. A portion of diced fruit fills half a cup. If the fruit is green grapes, a half-cup would be filled by about (a) 10; (b) 15; (c) 20.

5. A medium potato is about the size of (a) a computer mouse; (b) a matchbox car; (c) a light bulb.

6. For a portion of Brussels sprouts, which would come to half a cup, you would need (a) 4; (b) 8; (c) 12.

7. Two tablespoons of olive oil would more or less fill (a) a shot glass; (b) a thimble; (c) a Dixie Cup.

8. Two tablespoons of peanut butter could make a ball the size of (a) a marble; (b) a tennis ball; (c) a ping pong ball.

9. There are eight servings in a loaf of Entenmann's Raspberry Danish Twist. A serving in this case is the width of (a) one finger; (b) two fingers; (c) four fingers.

10. A medium apple or orange is about the size of (a) a softball; (b) a tennis ball; (c) a large wiffle ball.

**Answers:**
1c. 2a. 3b. 4b. 5a. 6a. 7a. 8c. 9c. 10b.

Adapted from *Tufts University Diet & Nutrition Letter.*

A number of masters began by weighing or measuring nearly every calorie-containing item they ate, just to get a feel for how much they were eating. (To do this, you'll need a good food scale, a set of measuring spoons and a set of measuring cups.) Some used the "Nutrition Facts" panel on packaged foods to guide portions, weighing or measuring the exact serving size indicated on the label.

Measuring all your food constantly, however, is not only tedious but impractical. *The good news is that most masters stop measuring once they get the hang of judging proper portion sizes.* Only about 1 out of 10 continues to measure on a regular basis; a number do so periodically. Now that JoAnna L. feels she knows what a "well-balanced but not overloaded meal" should consist of, she weighs and measures protein foods only one day a week. "In this way, my eyes don't start calling a 6-ounce portion of roast beef 3 ounces!" Some masters will again become more careful about weighing and measuring if their weight starts to creep up.

When planning portion sizes for the various food groups, keep in mind these servings, which are taken primarily from the Food Guide Pyramid, recommendations for healthy eating from the government.

◆ **Grain foods—bread, cereal, rice and pasta:** The recommended number of daily servings for foods in this category is 6 to 11 a day (6 servings are plenty for most women, 9 for most men). That may sound like a lot, but a serving is considered just 1 slice of bread; ½ cup of cooked cereal, rice or pasta; 1 ounce of dry cereal; ½ English muffin, hot dog or hamburger roll or bagel; 3 graham cracker squares; 5 slices of melba toast or 6 saltines or a 4-to-5-inch pancake.

◆ **Vegetables and fruits:** Try to have *at least* 5 servings a day. A serving of cooked vegetables or nonleafy raw vegetables is considered ½ cup; for leafy raw vegetables, a serving is 1 cup. (Leafy salad greens, like spinach and lettuce, are considered "free" foods that you can eat as often as you like.) A serving of fruit is considered 1 medium whole fruit, ½ cup canned or cut-up fresh fruit or ¾ cup (6 ounces) juice.

♦ **Milk products:** Your goal should be to try to have 2 to 3 servings a day. A portion is considered 1 cup of milk, 8 ounces of yogurt or 1½ to 2 ounces of cheese. The masters favor nonfat, no-sugar-added versions of these foods.

Interestingly, taste tests conducted by the Center for Science in the Public Interest revealed that when consumers were presented with milk of varying fat levels but not told which one they were drinking, few were able to taste the difference.

♦ **Meats, fish and poultry:** Nutrition experts recommend that portion sizes not exceed 2 to 3 ounces, cooked. Three ounces is about the size of a deck of cards or an average-sized woman's palm. In general, 4 ounces of boneless, skinless, trimmed raw flesh will net 3 ounces after cooking. If you're wondering how to "count" bone-in chicken, you'd get about 3 ounces of meat from any of the following (cooked, skinless): ½ of a whole chicken breast, 2 thighs or 2 drumsticks. (While it's not as critical to eat such tiny portion sizes for skinless poultry breast or seafood, it's generally recommended that we pay attention to amounts of all protein foods.) Other foods that count as 1 ounce of meat include: ½ cup of cooked legumes, 2 tablespoons peanut butter, 1 egg or ¼ cup cottage cheese.

♦ **Fats, oils and sweets:** There are no recommended amounts for these foods, other than to "use sparingly." A tablespoon of most fats has about 100 calories; a tablespoon of sugar has 45 calories. Label reading can help you figure out whether these items are worth the calories. Connye Z. says, "If it's something I really want, I'll probably get it anyway. But when the company started putting labels on cream horns, which I used to sometimes buy, I decided not to eat them anymore. They're good, but they're not *that* good!"

# READ THE LABEL

WHEN YOU SEE LABELS SUGGESTING better-for-you versions of products, use the "Nutrition Facts" panel to determine whether they really are. Some foods, such as fat-free pretzels and fig bars, are nothing special, since the original versions have very little fat to begin with. Here's what the jargon means when you see fat- and calorie-related claims on labels:

| If the label says: | It means the product has: |
|---|---|
| Reduced-fat, less fat | at least 25 percent less fat than the product with which it's being compared |
| Low-fat | no more than 3 grams of fat per serving |
| Low-calorie | no more than 40 calories per serving |
| Lite, light | at least one-third less calories, half the fat or half the sodium of the regular product |
| Fat-free | less than 0.5 gram of fat per serving |
| Calorie-free | less than 5 calories per serving |

Unfortunately, you cannot entirely trust package labels. For instance, products from small companies, like those individually packaged muffins or cookies you can pick up at convenience stores, can be mislabeled for weight, so you're getting more calories than you think. (Such products are not required to have nutrition labels unless they make health claims.) A recent study in the *Journal of the American Dietetic Association* found that for all but 2 of 19 such products, the actual measured weight exceeded the weight given on the label—often by as much as 20 to 25 percent. If you use such foods regularly, it's probably wise to weigh them yourself so you know how much you're really getting.

# A Low-Fat Portion Is Still a Portion

IKE DON, SOME MASTERS LEARNED THE HARD WAY that being mindful of portions is important even when those portions are low-fat or fat-free. Master Patsy K. avoids fat-free sweets for the following reason: "I have found that fat-free products do not work for me. I think it might be that word 'FREE'—I see it, and I think it means free to eat as much as I want of it." This phenomenon is known as "fat-free amnesia syndrome," according to Ruth Carpenter, M.S., R.D., of the Cooper Institute for Aerobics Research in Dallas. "It's when people forget that foods with little or no fat *do* provide calories."

The low-fat label may also trick us into eating more throughout the day, according to a study conducted at Monell Chemical Senses Center in Philadelphia. The research showed that when individuals were told their lunches were lower in fat than normal fare, they then consumed significantly more calories and fat at other times of the day than when they were told the lunches were high-fat. (Unbeknownst to the participants, the fat content of all the lunches was actually the same.) According to investigator Richard Mattes, Ph.D., R.D., "When people think they're eating low-fat foods, they may feel entitled to be more liberal with both calories and fat at other times without adverse consequences." Similar findings reported in the *Journal of the American Dietetic Association* showed that women who received yogurt labeled "low-fat" before a buffet-type meal ate more calories during the meal than when they were given yogurt that had about the same calories but was labeled "high-fat."

*Given two similar products with the same number of calories, it is usually healthier to choose the one with less fat.* Just don't kid yourself that you can eat all you want and keep your weight down. Be aware, too, that it's not just processed low-fat snack foods and desserts that can add up—so can naturally low-fat choices like rice and pasta. For example, a 2-cup serving of cooked spaghetti has more than 400 calories.

*The bottom line is that even when following a low-fat diet, you still have to cut back on calories if you want to lose weight. And you must keep watching calories if you want to keep weight off.*

# Drink More, Drink Less

Water drinking seems to help many masters take charge of their full buttons; 2 out of 3 indicated that they make a concerted effort to drink water to control their weight. Don Mauer says, "I drink gallons of bottled spring water. It tastes good, and it's refreshing."

Obesity expert James O. Hill, Ph.D., of the University of Colorado Health Sciences Center, theorizes: "Water does nothing metabolically that I know of, but I suspect it has satiety value—it makes you feel fuller, less hungry." And that's what a number of masters indicate—it helps them limit the amount they eat.

Don has another interesting theory about why water drinking helps: "I think obese people tend to misread thirst for hunger." Leslie S. concurs: "I've learned that when I think I'm hungry, I'm often just thirsty." Patsy K. adds, "When I get hungry between meals, I think I'm not really hungry. Water helps that feeling pass."

A number of masters drink diet soda. Shifting away from regular soda can save a ton of calories for heavy users like Emil R., who, at 335 pounds, used to drink "2,000 calories of Coke per day." Now weighing 220 pounds, he has Diet Coke and puts Equal in his coffee rather than sugar.

Cutting back on alcohol appears to be yet another way some masters put a clamp on how much food they eat. Diane J. says, "I limit alcoholic beverages to only once or twice a week, because they tend to make me overeat." Beth W. says they have the same effect on her: "I very seldom have alcohol, because it makes me hungry." Not only does alcohol tend to make some people relax with food control, it's fattening—with 7 calories per gram, alcohol comes close to fat, with its 9 calories per gram.

# Be Consistent

JUST AS ALCOHOL CAN SWAY YOU to let down your guard with food, so can erratic eating. The masters made this clear in their answers to my question, "How are your eating habits different than they were when you were heavy?" *They commonly responded that they no longer eat haphazardly and now go out of their way to eat regular meals and avoid skipping meals.* Consider the following "then" and "now" scenarios:

◆ "I never used to eat breakfast and sometimes skipped lunch. I now eat three meals a day and plan my snacks." —Lynda M. (36 pounds, 13 years)

◆ "When I was hungry, I ate all the time. It didn't matter if I had just finished dinner 30 minutes before. Now, I try to eat three meals a day and limit my snacks." —Peppi S. (27 pounds, 9 years)

◆ "I used to snack all day with only one main meal around 4:30 p.m. Now, I have three meals a day, spaced at least four hours apart, from the time I get up in the morning." —Maxine D. (39 pounds, 12 years)

While most masters eat three meals a day, many with planned snacks in between, some are grazers. Ann Q. (47 pounds, 7 years) has discovered, "I am not a three-meals-per-day person but, rather, do much better grazing on small quantities throughout the day." Diane J. (43 pounds, 5 years) eats a number of "mini-meals," as well as one main planned meal. She explains, "I try to eat something at least every three hours so I am not ever superhungry."

Like Don Mauer, who began eating breakfast when he started on his new way of eating, a number of masters stress the importance of breakfast. Joanne F. (80 pounds, 8 years) says, "Eating breakfast is a big change and is essential to keep me on track." Research supports her: A study on moderately obese women published in the *American Journal of Clinical Nutrition* showed that compared with nonbreakfast-eaters, those who ate breakfast tended to eat fewer impulsive snacks throughout the day and to eat more nutritionally balanced meals that were lower in fat.

*The critical message from the masters is, whether you eat several meals a day or graze throughout, you need to develop a daily routine—one that gives you consistency in your eating habits.*

You may be thinking that all of this planning, portioning and scheduling is more trouble than it's worth. The truth is that it does take some effort—especially in the beginning. But masters like Karen H. will tell you that the payback *is* worth it. Yes, she eats less often, eats slowly and always leaves something on her plate. What does she get in return? Besides being 92 pounds lighter, she exclaims, "I look at myself in the mirror each morning and feel great. But most of all, I can play and participate with my three boys!"

## CHAPTER FOUR

Food Secret #4:

# If You Want It, Have It

"Once I start, I can't stop."
"There's no way I can eat just one."
"I feel so guilty whenever I eat sweets."
"After I ate one, I figured I might as well eat
the whole bag . . ."

SUCH CONFESSIONS AND GRIEVANCES are all too common for dieters who lose weight and gain it back—but not the masters. Over and over, I heard comments such as, "I eat what I want" and "I allow myself treats." *In other words, if the masters want it, they have it. They have broken free of the deprivation syndrome—the feeling that you can't eat tempting foods, and when you do, you feel so guilty that you punish yourself by eating even more.* On the other hand, the masters know when to stop—they have control systems for tempting foods so they don't go overboard. How do *you* get to the point where you can eat what you want without remorse and feel satisfied with "just one," knowing full well you can have more tomorrow?

## Patsy K.'s Story

WHEN I ASK PATSY K., "How did you figure out what foods you could eat once you got down to your weight goal?" she responds, "I allowed myself a dessert every night; after all, I was used to eating sweets all day and night. If you entirely give up the foods that you have the most problems with, you will never learn how to eat them in moderation." After 19 years of being a master and 99 pounds lighter than her all-time high, she still has ice cream almost every night—and it's not always low-fat.

Patsy's weight problem began when she was in third grade. "My mom tried to help me cut back, but I recall sneaking out to get bread and crackers after the others went to bed."

She has "lost count" of all the times she tried to lose weight, using pills and putting herself on "starvation" diets, but binge eating always caused her to gain back even more. "I ate continuously, snacking on cookies, doughnuts and cakes until they were gone. I even woke up in the middle of the night and would eat ice cream, pudding, cereal or whatever was easy to grab. It was nothing for me to eat a half-gallon of ice cream, even if I didn't like the flavor."

She recalls being at a party one time after she had just lost 20 pounds, about to eat the dessert she had been served. "A thin woman said to me, 'I don't believe you're going to eat that—you just lost 20 pounds. You're going to gain it all back.' She was right—I did."

Her final four-year journey to lose began after she saw her doctor for a health problem and discovered that her weight had soared to 242 pounds. She decided to try TOPS (Take Off Pounds Sensibly), where the speaker emphasized the importance of losing weight without starving yourself. "I went home that night and realized that if I was going to lose weight and keep it off, I was going to have to change the way I eat. I decided to eat what I fixed for the family."

Before they went to bed, her four children always had a snack. Patsy joined them, allowing herself a daily treat, usually ice cream in a small custard cup. "I kept telling myself, 'You can have it again tomorrow and still lose weight.' When I used to try to give up ice cream completely, I would eventually eat the whole container. I just knew I couldn't give it up for the rest of my life."

For the first several months, Patsy weighed and measured food, wrote down everything she ate and used a calorie-counter book. She also watched her bills from the supermarket and baked-goods store plummet as she bought fewer sweets. Her husband cleaned up after dinner so she didn't have to handle the leftovers. When he worked at night, Patsy would leave the table, then go back to clean up much later, after the leftovers had dried out, so she wouldn't be tempted to eat them. She also recalls, "I did anything I could to stay out of the kitchen. I volunteered to work at the school library, joined ceramics and learned to crochet. I read more."

Today, Patsy still has her ice cream just about every evening—almost always in a small bowl or cone to control the amount—and occasionally allows herself a few bites during the day, "to satisfy the urge." She stresses the importance of never skipping a meal, particularly breakfast, which is typically cereal with skim milk and some fruit, such as strawberries, sliced banana or raisins, or one egg plus one egg white. She also has a cup of coffee with cream and sugar. Midmorning, she might have some juice or a piece of fruit. A typical lunch would be water-packed tuna on top of a mixed raw-vegetable salad with low-fat or fat-free dressing, along with some crackers or pretzels and either a glass of water or four ounces of real Coke. In the afternoon, Patsy's snack might consist of animal crackers and another piece of fruit. An everyday dinner for her is a plain baked potato, chicken breast grilled with seasoned salt or a combination of other spices, some green beans with onion powder and some iced tea or a little Coke. Then, just before bedtime, she treats herself.

# No More Forbidden Foods

PATSY'S STORY DEMONSTRATES yet another way the masters get themselves to keep doing what they do—if they want something, they have it. *Here's how to look at it: When you know you can have treat foods, it can provide the impetus for continuing to eat low-fat foods, keeping up with your exercise and watching the amount you eat.* "What made the difference for me was learning to eat all the things I like in a moderate amount," Patsy says. By contrast, she attributes previous failures to denying herself favorite foods.

Although a recent American Dietetic Association Survey of American Dietary Habits found that 3 out of 4 people believe there are "good" foods and "bad" foods, *breaking away from good food/bad food thinking has been a critical change for many masters.* As Ann F. adjusted to her 220-pound weight loss, she recalls, "I included food I like. I took away the taboo of 'forbidden foods.' " And Joanne F. says, "I knew that I would eventually have to learn how to handle my favorite but not-so-healthy foods, so I started planning occasional treats like fries and nachos when I got close to my goal."

When I asked the masters how they deal with food cravings, their number-one response was, "I have a little." Well over half indicated that they have a regular nondiet dessert at least once or twice a month; 80 of them said they do so at least once or twice a week. And when I asked the masters how they cope with "problem" foods, over and over I heard comments about how they allow themselves treats—but in moderation. After all, who would want to go through life *never* eating another ice cream cone, piece of chocolate or potato chip? From magazine covers to TV commercials to supermarket aisles filled with delectable foods, we're bombarded left and right with temptations to indulge. It's normal to want them, and it's okay to have them.

Margie M. urges, "Stop being so obsessed about what you can and cannot eat. There are no forbidden foods—just portion control." JoAnna L. concurs, "Because I don't have any forbidden foods any longer, I really don't have any problem foods. In the old days, it was cake doughnuts. I could go into our local quick-stop store and walk out with four of them. If I took the long way home, I could have them all wolfed down by the time I drove into our driveway and the bag stuffed under the front seat of the car for me to fish out later, when no one was around. But now that I've given myself permission to have a doughnut any time I want one—as long as I account for it in my food choices—I don't care if I have one or not."

Indeed, the very act of giving yourself permission to eat what you want can help with portion control. Marie C. (22 pounds, 5 years), a professional pastry chef who adores sweets, says: "I decide ahead of time that I'll eat a small amount and thoroughly savor it. I'll sit down, eat it slowly and enjoy and really taste every bite." Don Mauer, who for the first five years of maintenance denied himself chocolate, now keeps snack-sized Snickers bars in his refrigerator. "It's not a full-sized bar, so it's a controlled amount. But I can eat just one and know that there are nine more in the package. Because I removed the denial, I can now eat these foods."

As with other aspects of weight control, you have to find what works for you. While most masters comfortably handle tempting foods, a relatively small number feel a need to avoid them altogether—about 1 in 10 masters completely avoids sweets or desserts. For others, feeling at ease with treats did not happen immediately. Katie G. says, "It took some time to realize that I wouldn't wake up fat the next morning if I ate a meal *and* had my chocolate fix."

# No More Guilt, No More Deprivation

THE MESSAGE IS SIMPLE: *When you have treats, enjoy them. You don't have to feel guilty.* Karen S. (23 pounds, 18 years) says, "I've accepted the fact that I will always love certain foods and can have them and enjoy them on occasion." The "certain foods" for Karen are salty, crunchy items and some candies. "I allow myself to eat them, but in lesser quantities. I enjoy them rather than berating myself for eating them." Dorothy J. (40 pounds, 15 years) explains how she guiltlessly handles what could be, for many, a disastrous situation with tempting foods. "Since my husband and I own a bakery, customers often comment, 'How do you stay so trim working here?' My answer is, 'I don't eat goodies often, but when I do, I enjoy every bite!'" Shirley G., who's kept off 85 pounds for the better part of 20 years, adds, "There is nothing I completely avoid. That, to me, would be very depressing. I don't think I have as many cravings now that I eat a little of everything. Depriving yourself totally is not the key."

# DESTIGMATIZING SWEETS

IT'S A COMMON ASSUMPTION that sugar and other carbohydrates contribute to overeating and obesity. Yet according to a recent review of research studies on the question by Pennsylvania State University's Barbara Rolls, Ph.D., "There is little direct evidence that obese individuals eat excessive quantities of sweet foods." In fact, she points out that several studies suggest just the opposite: People who are thin tend to eat more sugar than those who are heavy.

In and of themselves, table sugar (sucrose) and corn syrup are no worse for you than so-called natural sugars from foods such as fruit. The body cannot distinguish between "natural" and added sugars. Because of the other nutrients in them, however, foods naturally containing sugar *do* tend to be more healthful than those with a lot of added sugars. Fruit, for instance, has fiber, vitamins and minerals that are lacking in "empty-calorie" sweets like candy, cake and cookies. Many high-sugar foods are also high in fat.

Other conditions erroneously linked to sugar consumption are diabetes and hyperactivity. There is no evidence that diabetes is caused by sugar consumption, and many people with diabetes can now include modest amounts of sugar in their diets, as long as they're under medical supervision. As for hyperactivity, the recently released government-sponsored Dietary Guidelines for Americans states: "Scientific evidence indicates that diets high in sugars do not cause hyperactivity." Some studies suggest that sugar may actually have a calming effect.

The Dietary Guidelines recommend doing what most of the masters seem to do: "Choose a diet moderate in sugars."

# No More "Eating Around" What You Really Want

**P**ATSY K. EXPLAINS WHAT HAPPENS when she tries to fight a craving: "If I deny myself, I wind up eating lots of different things and then giving in to the craving after all. I could have saved myself a lot of calories if I would have just satisfied my craving. Sometimes, just a taste is all I need, and then I can go on." Patsy is talking about the common problem of "eating all around what you really want."

Ann Rae A. says, "If I want chocolate, I no longer try to put off the feeling by ignoring it or trying to eat something else instead. I found that I was eating too much other stuff, and when I would finally 'break down,' I would totally lose it and eat too much."

# Develop a Control System for Tempting Foods

**N**OW THAT I'VE TOLD YOU *how important it is for most maintainers to allow themselves treats, I'm going to turn around and tell you how important it is to come up with a system for limiting them.* Although the masters can and do eat tempting foods, they accept the fact that there will *never* be a point in time at which they can eat whatever they want, whenever they want—and that's true for the vast majority of people on this earth! If you pay close attention to the habits of people who have never had a weight problem, I'd venture to say you'll find very few who exhibit no restraint when it comes to food. One study, published in the *American Journal of Clinical Nutrition*, compared women who had lost weight and kept it off with women who had never been heavy. Researchers found that the women who had always been slim consciously worked to stay that way; they had a number of the same habits as the women who had lost weight. The truth is, you can't have your cake and eat it too—at least not all of it!

*To develop a control system, first you have to identify your own personal high-temptation foods.* What tempts one person may not particularly interest another, and it's important to be aware of exactly what foods entice you the most: Simply make a list of your favorite items. Sweets fall into the problem-food category for 3 out of 4 masters. As JoAnn L. puts it, "My problem foods are probably the same as for 95 percent of all people dieting: I love sweets—especially pastries and pies." Like many masters, Valerie D. says her sweet weakness is "chocolate—anything made of chocolate."

The next highest category of temptation for the masters comes from snack-type items like chips and other salty foods. For instance, Nancy K.'s downfall is potato chips and nuts. Finally, quite a few masters identified specific foods like pizza, bread, cheese, meats and peanut butter.

# Triage to Prevent Temptation

Once you've compiled your list of high-temptation foods, it helps to triage, grouping them into categories depending on the degree to which you feel you can control them. Patsy K., for instance, can obviously control her desire for ice cream. But of Doritos and potato chips she says, "I avoid eating the first one."

When Linda W. (44 pounds, 8 years) craves pizza, she is "satisfied by a lunch at Pizza Hut and three pieces," but when it comes to foods like nuts and chips, "I dare not start nibbling on them between meals. For me, it would be kind of like falling off the booze wagon. So I just don't start."

The masters use control tactics depending on how well they feel they can handle particular foods:

## Tactic #1

**Don't even start.** Although most masters allow themselves treats, more than half indicated that there are certain foods they completely avoid. Dorothy J. notes, "Chocolate is a 'trigger' food, so I don't have it around."

## Tactic #2

**Out of sight, out of mind.** It's straightforward: If tempting foods are not around, you can't eat them. Connye Z. abides by the rule: "I don't buy things that I know are my weaknesses, at least not on a regular basis." *About 2 out of every 3 masters keep problem foods out of the house or out of sight.* Liane F., who has trouble with peanut butter, says, "I put it far back in the refrigerator so I don't see it."

Bob W. remarks, "I don't have problem foods in the house—I go out for them. As W.C. Fields said, 'I can resist anything except temptation!' I *know* myself."

## Tactic #3

**Use stopgap measures.** A number of masters find ways to control the amount of treat foods they eat at any one time. When he has the urge for yogurt-covered pretzels and chocolate-covered peanuts, Emil R. buys 30-to-50-cents' worth from a bulk bin. Thalia A. makes it a rule never to eat potato chips "unsupervised, meaning in secret." If she were alone, she might eat chips indiscriminately but feels restraint when she's with others. Lynda M. has discovered that it's not the end of the world to dispose of food that might turn out to be a problem for her. "I once threw out a chocolate-cherry pound cake after my husband and I had enjoyed some of it."

## Tactic #4

**Don't food-shop when hungry.** Nearly half the masters, including Patsy K., say they use this technique. Rose B. affirms, "If I buy groceries in the afternoon, I always get Hershey's Hugs. Now, I buy groceries right after breakfast, when I'm not hungry and it isn't 'candy time.'" Kathy G., who has a penchant for sweets, avoids supermarket aisles stocked with candy and cookies.

## Tactic #5

**Set aside treat days.** A number of masters permit themselves to have their tempting foods only on weekends. Joy C., who loves rich pies and cakes, states, "I allow myself a treat over the weekend, but one normal piece."

# Tactic #6

**Make trade-offs.** In other words, if you have a treat, forgo something else. If Connye Z. is going to a party or a restaurant, she saves up for it, eating less during the day so she can treat herself that night.

# Tactic #7

**Substitute a reduced-fat or low-calorie version of the food you're craving.** More than half the masters indicated that they have a reduced-fat dessert at least once or twice a week. For instance, Lynda M. says she keeps a check on her love of chocolate by "using low-fat, low-calorie products—pudding, cookies and frozen yogurt." Karen S. says that when she has a craving for something salty, she might have "something similar, but in a low-fat version—for example, reduced-fat Wheatables or Bugles instead of potato chips or corn chips."

*At least some of the time, some masters substitute a food healthier than the item they're longing for.* When Chuck B. has a craving, he has "pretzels, popcorn, veggies or fruit. I feel better after these snacks, and most are more refreshing." Kevin E. remarks, "I usually eat rice or pasta when craving a cheeseburger. I eat popcorn when craving potato chips." Jane Brody's favorite snacks include frozen yogurt, unsalted pretzels and hot-air-popped popcorn—three snacks the masters often mentioned.

The masters seem to find that popcorn and pretzels take care of the craving for high-fat, salty and crunchy snacks, such as chips and cheese curls, many of which get more than half of their calories from fat. Patsy K. states, "Air-popped popcorn is great for snacking. It gives you the satisfaction you need when you get the munchies." Cam L., who has a weakness for nuts, says, "I am able to substitute pretzels sometimes." When satisfying your "salt tooth," be careful to check labels, however, because a number of popcorn products and a few specialty pretzels are quite high in fat.

The masters have come up with some great low-fat ideas to heighten the flavor of air-popped popcorn, such as mixing air-popped and microwave popcorn together, adding a little high-quality olive oil and curry powder, sprinkling with some Parmesan cheese or spraying with a light coating of nonstick spray and adding salt. (For more ideas, see the opposite page.)

# Eating Thin for Life Popcorn Recipes

I N THE FOLLOWING RECIPES, spray popcorn lightly with butter-flavored nonstick cooking spray to help seasonings stick. Sprinkle with half the seasonings and toss, spray lightly again, add remaining seasonings and toss. Season with salt, if desired.

To make 4 cups reduced-fat popcorn on the stovetop, cook 2½ tablespoons popcorn in 1 teaspoon vegetable oil. This will add 43 calories plus 5 grams of fat to any of the first eight recipes and 86 calories and 10 grams of fat to the Popcorn Balls.

| Recipe | Ingredients | Serves | NUTRIENTS/SERVING* | |
| --- | --- | --- | --- | --- |
| | | | Calories | Fat (grams) |
| Ranch Popcorn | 4 cups hot popcorn | 1 | 148 | 1 |
| | 1 tablespoon dry Ranch dressing mix | | | |
| Cheese Popcorn | 4 cups hot popcorn | 1 | 179 | 5 |
| | 2 tablespoons Parmesan cheese | | | |
| Nacho Cheese Popcorn | 4 cups hot popcorn | 1 | 173 | 4 |
| | 2 tablespoons grated American cheese food | | | |
| | ⅛ teaspoon cayenne pepper | | | |
| Holiday Popcorn | 4 cups hot popcorn | 1 | 154 | 1 |
| | 1 teaspoon red sugar crystals | | | |
| | 1 teaspoon green sugar crystals | | | |

* Nutrition information based on 4 cups air-popped popcorn. Cooking spray not included in analysis.

| Recipe | Ingredients | Serves | NUTRIENTS/SERVING* | |
|---|---|---|---|---|
| | | | Calories | Fat (grams) |
| Mexican Popcorn | 4 cups hot popcorn | 1 | 137 | 1 |
| | ½ tablespoon dry taco seasoning | | | |
| | cayenne pepper | | | |
| Italian Popcorn | 4 cups hot popcorn | 1 | 128 | 1 |
| | 1 teaspoon Italian seasoning, crushed | | | |
| | ¼ teaspoon garlic salt | | | |
| Oriental Popcorn | 4 cups hot popcorn | 1 | 123 | 1 |
| | shakes of soy sauce | | | |
| | ⅛ teaspoon five-spice powder | | | |
| Cinnamon-Sugar Popcorn | 4 cups hot popcorn | 1 | 160 | 1 |
| | 1 teaspoon cinnamon | | | |
| | 2 teaspoons sugar | | | |
| Popcorn Balls | 3 tablespoons margarine | 8 | 182 | 5 |
| | 1 (10-ounce) bag marshmallows | | | |
| | food coloring (optional) | | | |
| | 8 cups popcorn | | | |

**To make popcorn balls:** Melt margarine in a bowl in the microwave or in a pan on the stove. Add marshmallows and continue to heat until melted. Stir until smooth. Mix in food coloring, if using. Pour over popcorn and stir to coat. Spray hands with nonstick cooking spray. Working quickly, form into balls. Cool on wax paper.

As far as frozen yogurts are concerned, the masters find they make great substitutes for ice cream and other sweets. Whitney V. states, "I always need a goodie, so thank God for frozen yogurt!" The list of frozen yogurts and "light" ice cream products keeps growing, but check labels, because some products are quite a bit higher in fat and calories than others.

# Handle Cravings Without Eating

A LTHOUGH THE MASTERS' NUMBER-ONE WAY to deal with food cravings is to give in, in moderation, many of them also mentioned alternative ways of handling cravings.

♦ **Wait it out.** Sometimes, cravings do go away if you wait a while. As Joanne F. explains, "I remember that it will pass." Jim V. agrees: "I wait about 20 to 30 minutes, and cravings usually pass."

♦ **Talk to yourself.** It can help to try to sort out whether there's an emotional reason for your craving. Joanne F. explains that when she craves something, "I try to understand why I'm craving it." She adds, "If I choose to have it, I try and remember it was my choice." Ann F. elaborates, "I try to figure out what I'm feeling: anxiety? fatigue? depression? I try to deal with that in other ways."

♦ **Have a no-calorie beverage.** When she has a craving, Lynda M. combines several techniques: "I drink water and wait 15 to 20 minutes. If I still crave it, I have a small amount and remind myself that I *know* what this tastes like."

# The Problem of Binge Eating: A Craving Out of Control

**N**EARLY HALF THE MASTERS feel they were binge eaters in the past. No one knows how many people suffer from binge eating, but according to the National Institutes of Health, it is estimated that about 10 to 15 percent of mildly obese individuals in self-help or commercial weight-loss programs have "binge-eating disorder." It is more common in severely obese people. The difference between binge eating and plain old overeating or giving in to a craving has to do not only with the *amount* you eat at any one time but also with the *degree of control* you feel over the situation. Psychiatrists and psychologists consider a binge to be a situation in which you consume, within a relatively short time period, a much larger volume of food than most people would eat, and you feel you cannot stop or control what you're eating. When such binges occur frequently, a person likely has binge-eating disorder. Here's how some masters described their binges:

♦ "I would starve all day, and then once I was alone at night, I'd eat one thing after another: a quart of ice milk, a dozen cookies, a pound of licorice." —Becky M. (36 pounds, 13 years)

♦ "I would binge three to five times a week. I might eat a whole pizza, three or four candy bars, whole carrot cakes, bags of potato chips, half-gallons of ice cream." —Bob W. (246 pounds, 23 years)

♦ "I might sit down and eat a three-to-four-pound roast." —Ron K. (61 pounds, 7 years)

♦ "I would binge at least weekly, most often after coming off some very restrictive diet. I would eat a big bag of chips, Doritos, a quart of ice cream, two to three candy bars and buttered popcorn." —Ann F. (220 pounds, 11 years)

# Putting the Lid on Binge Eating

How did the masters who used to binge overcome their problem?

**Some masters stressed the importance of not depriving themselves.** Patsy K. found that it helped when she figured out that she could eat the so-called forbidden foods and still maintain her weight. Cathy B. adds that *not* denying herself foods she really likes helps her to "never feel a real need to overindulge or binge to compensate."

**Others mentioned the necessity of not letting themselves get too hungry.** When Lynda C. began having regular meals throughout the day, she felt as though she was eating a great deal but soon lost 10 pounds. Don Mauer adds, "If you eat normal-sized meals several times a day, you have a tendency not to be ravenous."

**Many masters now fill up on healthy or low-fat foods when they feel like binge eating.** Peppi S. states, "When I feel a binge coming on, I only 'binge' on fat-free snacks. And after the first few handfuls, the binge usually subsides."

**Quite a few masters emphasized how important it is not to keep problem foods in the house.** Alyce keeps "only 'okay' foods around that I can't binge on if I tried. Who is going to binge on lettuce?"

**Many stressed that it is helpful to come up with an alternative activity when they feel the need to binge.** Evelyn C. reads a good book or story; Virginia L. writes, calls a friend or reads.

**Some masters find that exercising is of value.** Arlene Z. states, "Exercise has helped a lot—walking allows time to put life into perspective."

**But the masters' top technique for putting a lid on bingeing is talking to themselves and trying to figure out why they feel like going on a binge.** Katie G. explains, "I recognize my hungers for what they are and feed them as needed. When my stomach growls, I eat.

# PROGRAMS FOR BINGE-EATING DISORDER

**Arbor Counseling Center**
110 N. Essex Avenue
Narberth, PA 19072
(610) 664-5858

**Behavioral Medicine**
Stanford University
  School of Medicine
Department of Psychiatry
401 Quarry Street
Stanford, CA 94305
(415) 723-5868

**Behavioral Medicine
  Research Clinic**
Baylor College of
  Medicine
6535 Fannin Street,
  MS F700
Houston, TX 77030
(713) 789-5757

**Binge-Eating Program**
Western Psychiatric
  Institute and Clinic
3811 O'Hara Street
Pittsburgh, PA 15213
(412) 624-2823

**Eating Disorder Research
  Program**
University of Minnesota
2701 University Avenue,
  S.E., Suite 206
Minneapolis, MN 55414
(612) 627-4494

**Eating Disorders Clinic**
New York State Psychiatric
  Institute
Columbia Presbyterian
  Medical Center
722 W. 168th Street,
  Unit #98
New York, NY 10032
(212) 960-5739/5746

**Rutgers Eating
  Disorders Clinic**
Rutgers University
41 Gordon Road
Piscataway, NJ 08854
(908) 445-2292

**Department of
  Psychology**
Yale Center for Eating
  and Weight Disorders
P.O. Box 208205
New Haven, CT
  06520-8205
(203) 432-4610

*Updated from "Binge Eating Disorder," National Institute of Diabetes & Digestive & Kidney Diseases, National Institutes of Health Publication No. 94-3589, 1993.*

When I'm feeling down or sad, I call a friend or read a book or hop on my rollerblades—or drink a few beers, cry a little and go to sleep! When my soul feels empty, I pick up a pen and write out what's going on inside of me."

# Cut Your Losses

TO BE SURE, the masters are not always 100 percent in control of tempting foods and their cravings, but they don't punish themselves when they slip back into old ways. *In short, they cut their losses and move on.* Lynda M. says, "I've learned to forgive myself when I blow my eating plan and get back on track as soon as I can. The 'old' me would have used that as an excuse to keep on eating. I've learned I can rectify mistakes, and one overindulgence isn't going to make me gain back the 39 pounds I lost." This is a critical difference from many people who regain lost weight—the masters give themselves permission to be human and don't allow occasional lapses to become a trigger for weight gain.

Patsy K. explains, "There are times when I go over my 1,800-calorie limit with ice cream or other desserts. I do feel a little guilt, but then I forgive myself and go on. You have to be able to put it behind you."

*The bottom line for most masters when it comes to tempting foods is that if they want them, they have them in moderation. But when moderation doesn't work, they forgive themselves and move on.* Take the advice of Katie G., whose ability to enjoy treats and find pleasures in life other than food has enabled her to keep off 30 pounds for 7 years: "Lighten up mentally! Satisfy yourself and have fun. If eating a Snickers bar will make you smile, then have one, lick your fingers and go on to something else—not something edible, though. Read a book, rollerblade, chat on the phone, make love, and have at least one good belly laugh a day!"

## CHAPTER FIVE

Food Secret #5:

# Don't Let the Tough Times Get You Down

*When it comes to your weight-loss efforts, does this sound familiar?*

I did fine until . . .

. . . I went on vacation.

. . . I had my first baby.

. . . I went to that wedding.

. . . I got PMS.

. . . evening came, and I turned on the TV.

. . . I quit smoking.

. . . my mother said, "Have some pie; you're getting too thin."

. . . my skinny husband got out a bag of chips.

IT CAN BE A SINGLE EVENT or an accumulation of challenges that throws even the most well-intentioned slimmed-down person off track. Sometimes, it's a seemingly minor event, such as going to a special restaurant or watching a family member enjoy a favorite food. Other times, it's a milestone, such as going through a divorce, having a baby or experiencing a death in the family. In this chapter, the masters share how they survive the tough times—from nighttime yearnings and premenstrual cravings to social events with tempting foods. They describe how they got through pregnancies, quitting smoking and losing loved ones. They also tell how they deal with individuals who push food on them and how they cope with family members whose eating habits are different from theirs. The masters share ideas for managing your own challenges—be they large or small—without gaining back your weight.

# Joanne F.'s Story

JOANNE F. CAUGHT MY ATTENTION when she appeared in a photograph in *Life* magazine dressed in nothing but a pair of her former size-20 pants, her now size-8 body taking up just half of them. In the photo, she appears happy and carefree. In conversation, she gives every indication of being a "together" 33-year-old. She exclaims, "I now weigh less than I did in the sixth grade." But both before and after her 80-pound weight loss, Joanne survived some tough times that she did not let stand in her way.

From eighth grade on, she notes, "at least once a year, I would lose 30 or 40 pounds and gain it back." You name the diet or diet program, and Joanne had tried it. When she wasn't dieting, Joanne says she ate mindlessly. The turning point came when she went through counseling to help her deal with the fact that she had been sexually abused as a child, beginning in second grade—exactly the time when she began to gain. She began to see that being overweight gave her "a secure place, protection and an excuse—I could blame almost everything on my weight. For my parents, food was the Band-Aid—if I was sad, the message was, 'Have something to eat.' "

She reached her goal weight of 130 in 1986 and soon opened up her own business, which she runs to this day with a partner. After coasting for several years, Joanne then hit an emotional roadblock and slowly regained 25 to 30 pounds. "People think that when the weight is gone, it is gone forever and that their problems will be gone too," she observes. But the scar was still there for Joanne, who had trouble accepting the fact that when she lost weight, men became interested in her. "I had never had to deal with sex or sexuality. I got desperate for my 'protection' back." Joanne finally realized that being overweight was more painful than the alternative, and she returned to Weight Watchers, which had helped her when she initially lost the weight.

She also came up with a list of reasons to lose, putting individual items on flash cards:

- I want to be able to run three miles.
- I want to look in the mirror and feel good about myself.
- I want to be healthy.

"Some of the cards were funny," she says. "For instance, because I had a friend who used to pinch the extra skin on my back, one card said, 'I don't want to be gripped anymore.'" She gave the cards to a few trusted friends who she knew wouldn't badger her. "If I was struggling or I asked them to, they would read a card to me," she explains. "To this day, one of them carries a card in his wallet and flashes it at me occasionally when I say something negative about my weight."

Like all other masters, Joanne is faced with day-to-day food challenges. Her tough time of day—when she's most tempted to overeat—is late at night. It became even tougher when she took on a second job as a caretaker of special-needs people several nights a week. At first, she found herself thinking, " 'I'll have more energy if I eat.' But it wasn't true." So after her charges are asleep, she keeps herself busy with some of her more mindless chores, such as paying bills or writing memos for her daytime job. When she's at home evenings, she tries not to stay up too late. Sometimes, she does crossword puzzles (easy ones so that she doesn't get frustrated), and she often saves a healthful snack like an apple for late at night. "I can't have a treat then—unless it's something like a single-serving Weight Watchers dessert—because I'm more vulnerable at that time and won't be able to stop."

Another challenge Joanne has learned to cope with is "the food pusher"—someone who can't take no for an answer. When Joanne began to lose weight, her mother feared she was becoming anorexic and insisted on making cookies for her, offering them to her with the words, "I made your favorite." After eating a small amount, Joanne learned to assert, "I'm full. This is enough for me." Other family members complained that Joanne was acting as though she was "too good" for them now that she was thin. (Most of them struggle with their weight.) When there was too much pressure, Joanne would hang up in the middle of phone conversations or threaten not to go home for visits. "I had to get across that this was important to me." Now that she's been a master for more than 8 years, she is good at simply saying, "No, thank you." Or she takes a little of what she's offered, then puts it down somewhere. She adds, "If I get food for a gift, I immediately give it away."

In addition to maintaining a vegetarian low-fat diet, Joanne is committed to exercise and does some sort of activity just about every day—usually walking, sometimes while using hand-held weights. She continues to go to Weight Watchers meetings at least once a month and doesn't hesitate to go back more frequently when she's having trouble.

She admits that it is still difficult for her to keep her weight down. "I am constantly aware of my issues with food," she says. "I will always have to monitor my choices." But with time and acceptance, she notes, "the challenge has become less consuming."

Joanne keeps a "before" photo of herself by the scale in her bathroom. "It helps make the struggle worth it." She also discarded her old clothes, all the way up to size 22. "I got rid of those safety cushions that I could go back to." Finally, Joanne keeps herself going by taking advantage, whenever she can, of opportunities to talk about her success—from Weight Watchers contests to her *Life* magazine appearance. "Going public keeps me on track. I don't want someone from *Life* to come back to me 10 years from now and find that I've gained the weight back!"

As Joanne points out, losing weight doesn't make all problems go away. Life may still dish up unhappiness. People and personalities may still get in your way. Your old habits—like nighttime eating—may rear their ugly heads from time to time. And even the happy times, like births and weddings, may pose a challenge at maintenance. *But the masters have made the choice: Rather than throw up their hands and give up, they've decided to weather the tough times without gaining back their weight.*

Now that they're well into maintenance, the masters have lots of creative ways for handling the tough times. Sometimes, they have setbacks and start to regain, as Joanne did, but they rally to stay on top of their success. Here's how you can learn from the masters for those "what-do-you-do-when" times.

# You Hit Your Tough Time of Day?

L IKE JOANNE, almost all the masters indicated that they have a time of day when it's tough to control their eating. The most common "tough time" is after supper—about 1 in 3 masters has difficulty then. Next comes the afternoon, followed by suppertime and then late at night. (Very few masters have problems earlier in the day.)

Ann F. deals with her desire to eat in the evening by using the masters' most popular strategy—*do something other than eat.* She says, "I do something pleasurable, such as take a bath, do my nails or talk on the phone." Jim V. states, "I try to occupy my evening time with something constructive that I enjoy—a good book, a good movie, some computer work at home or going out with friends to a non-eating function." A number of masters plan their exercise for their tough time of day.

Many masters make an effort to *have low-fat nutritious foods and/or beverages at that time.* For instance, Karen S., who has trouble around 4 p.m., says that if she can't get out of the house or out of the kitchen at that time, "I might make tea and have one decent snack. Occasionally, if I can get my act together, I'll have those peeled baby carrots around and eat lots of them with salsa or Dijon mustard." Beth W.'s game plan for dealing with her problem time (between work and supper) is, "Before I leave work, I try to eat a piece of fruit or something to fill me up. When I get home, I grab a can of pop to drink while I'm fixing supper." Some masters, like Kay D., profiled in Chapter One, reserve a treat food for their tough time of day. She explains, "I save a food to eat that really satisfies my urge, such as ice cream. I allocate myself a certain amount each night and look forward to it."

# 15 WAYS TO DEAL WITH YOUR TOUGH TIME OF DAY

Call a friend.
Go for a walk.
Get involved in a hobby.
Have a low-fat snack.
Save a treat for that time.
Drink a no-cal beverage.
Go to bed.
Make love.

Brush your teeth.
Stay out of the kitchen.
Sort out your feelings.
Turn off the TV.
Take a hot bath.
Read a great book or
    magazine article.
Get out of the house.

WHAT DO YOU DO WHEN . . .

# It's That Time of the Month?

LIKE NEARLY HALF OF THE OTHER FEMALE MASTERS, Joanne F. reports changes in her eating habits in relation to her menstrual cycle. The week before her period, Joanne "craves carbs" like bread, an urge that used to make her feel out of control. But now when she has her cravings, she simply looks at the calendar. When she finds that it's almost that time of the month, she says, "Mostly, I just acknowledge the craving. It's easier to control when I understand why. I just remember it will pass. But sometimes, I just eat!"

Actually, the most commonly craved foods the masters mention in conjunction with menstrual periods are sweets. Lynda C. declares, "I *crave* sugar when I'm premenstrual." Most women yearn for chocolate. But some, like Whitney V., crave "more starchy, salty things, like potato chips and pretzels."

Although there is some scientific evidence that women may need more calories—anywhere from 8 to 16 percent more—during the last two weeks of the menstrual cycle, just after ovulation, there is no explanation why certain women crave sweets, others salty foods. *The masters' advice about menstrual-related desires is to give in to them—within reason:*

- "I try not to be too rigid with myself. If I try too hard to fight it, I always lose, so I let myself have limited treats, knowing I won't feel that way the next week." —Vicki B. (61 pounds, 10 years)
- "I usually allow myself to have something sweet during the week before my period. It seems to help my mood too." —Peppi S. (27 pounds, 9 years)
- "I give in, in moderation. It makes me feel better—the acceptance of 'okay, I need salt and chocolate.' I'll retain fluid and gain two pounds, but in a week, the pounds and the cravings will be gone." —Ann Rae A. (100 pounds, 4 years)
- "I want to binge before my period. It is usually only one day, and I do give in. For example, I wanted pecan pie, but instead of eating the whole pie, I ate only a couple of bites, proving to myself that I am still in control." —Cindy P. (80 pounds, 12 years)

Indulging in moderation isn't the only way the masters cope. Lenna D. tries to eat more fruits and vegetables. Jennifer P., who yearns for chocolate the week before her period, says, "I try to reduce stress, relax, exercise, meditate and warn my family."

Some masters use exercise to counter menstrual cravings. "I do eat more," explains Karen H., "but I increase my exercise from two to three days per week to three to four days and do it for longer."

HAT DO YOU DO WHEN . . .

# Someone Pushes Food on You?

NANCY G. ADMITS, "It takes time to get past the comments, 'You're thin enough,' 'A little dessert won't hurt you,' 'How can you eat that many vegetables?' or 'It would be so much easier if you ate what everyone else does.'"

She is describing all-too-familiar comments from people who, knowingly or unknowingly, attempt to sabotage slimmed-down people.

# GREAT LINES FOR STOPPING FOOD PUSHERS IN THEIR TRACKS

## Be Assertive

◆ "I ask people if they would offer a cigarette to someone trying to stop smoking or a beer to someone trying to stop drinking. It works." —Wayne P. (120 pounds, 3 years)

◆ "If people persist, I ask them, 'Why is it so important to you that I eat it?'" —Emil R. (115 pounds, 9 years)

◆ "I tell them, 'I do not *want* any.' It gives me strength to say it aloud." —Alicia G. (145 pounds, 10 years)

## Use Humor

◆ "I say, 'I'm allergic to that—it makes me break out in fat.'" —Marie T. (43 pounds, 9 years)

◆ "I smile and say something stupid like, 'If I eat any more, I'll throw up all over your new Nike tennis shoes.'" —Katie G. (30 pounds, 7 years)

## Blame It on Your Health

◆ "Sometimes, if they press, I say, 'I've just been to the dentist, and I can't eat,' or 'My pancreas won't let me eat that.'" —Alyce (93 pounds, 20 years)

◆ "I tell them, 'I'm not feeling well.'" —Anna M. (32 pounds, 10 years)

◆ "I say, 'I have chronic food intolerance.' They aren't quite sure what that is, so they leave me alone." —Virginia L. (97 pounds, 4 years)

When I asked the masters how they go about handling food pushers, most of them indicated that *they politely decline the offer.* Marlene R. adds, "I just say, 'No, thank you' and feel proud when I say it." Chuck B.'s policy is, "I politely say, 'Thanks, but no thanks. I don't want to carry that old body around again.' I let them know my weight is how it is because I say no."

Like Chuck, some masters find it helps to make others aware of their weight-loss success. Celia G. explains, "I tell them about losing 40 pounds. They're usually impressed, can't believe it and stop pushing me." Karen H. tells food pushers, "Thank you, but I have worked hard to lose weight, and I choose not to cheat myself by gaining it back."

A number of masters might have a small amount of what the person is offering. Stephanie C.'s policy is, "If it's a special day, I will take a limited amount of no-no food." Maxine D. says, "If I want some, I'll take it and eat only what I want. Otherwise, I can get as rude as they are pushy."

Other masters say they're not hungry. Evelyn C. tells food pushers, "No, thank you, I've just eaten a huge lunch." Jane Brody might say, "It was really delicious, but I've had enough," or "Maybe I could take some home."

But when polite refusals don't work, some masters just get plain ornery when food is pushed on them. Dorothy C.'s position is, "No one can really pressure me to eat. If I let someone push food on me, it's because I want it and am using that as an excuse." *The masters make it clear that they don't let food pushers push them around.*

# Relationships Change?

WHILE CLOSE TO HALF OF THE MASTERS found that their relationships stayed much the same after they slimmed down, others felt that friends, relatives and even total strangers treated them differently. Stan J. says, "Some of my friends look up to me as an example of success, others point me out as a future failure, while still others accuse me of 'cheating' when I eat certain foods."

As Stan's experience so aptly illustrates, it's not all praise and glory from significant others when you lose weight.

## Dealing with the Negative

**Your friends may become jealous.** The most common negative changes in relationships described by the masters have to do with jealousy. Now that she's lost 111 pounds, Kay D. finds, "Many of my still-heavy friends shun me and try to sabotage my maintenance by saying, 'Oh, she will gain it back.' Some make excuses not to be with me."

**You may lose old food buddies.** Joanne F. used to have a group of friends who were all overweight. Their relationship was based on their common love of eating. But after she slimmed down, those friendships started to end. "I tried to say, 'No, I don't want the fries. I want Diet Coke, and I'm here to talk with you.' But it didn't work. Now, I base friendships on trying to know people rather than habits we have together."

Patsy B. observes, "Friends have difficulty eating with me. They feel bad eating fat with me around. I haven't lost friends, but they laugh off the way I live." Lolly D. adds, "Some of my friends still need to be reminded at times that I have to stick to these healthier changes even if they choose unhealthy foods. This continues to be one of the hardest things to accept: that people who claim to care the most do not support my efforts for a healthier lifestyle."

**Your spouse may be threatened.** While some spouses react with pride when their partners lose weight, others respond negatively. "It didn't take very long for my marriage to unravel when I lost the weight," remembers Alyce. Around the time that she met her goal, she recalls buying a gorgeous backless outfit to wear for her wedding-anniversary dinner. While Alyce was waiting for her then-husband to be impressed, he remarked, "Oh, that's cute," in an offhand manner, and the rest of the evening proceeded in an uncomfortable fashion. Alyce thinks her ex-husband's insecurities and his worries about increased male competition led to his repeated attempts to sabotage her efforts by making suggestions like, "Let's go out for pizza," when he knew she was trying to lose weight.

Jeff B. also believes that his marriage faltered because of his weight loss. At one point, his wife threatened to leave him because she felt he was getting too thin. "For the first time, I felt I was attractive to other women. I became more outgoing, flirty and interested in messing around, so I wasn't the same person."

It's critical to keep the lines of communication open, and it may be wise to get some professional counseling if you foresee yourself in similar circumstances.

## Now for the Positive

**You may acquire more friends, better friends.** Because of positive changes in themselves, a number of masters find they now enjoy a wider social circle. Joanne F. says, "Mostly, I have gained friends; I'm now more outgoing and social." Since losing weight, Faye R. finds that her relationships have improved because she is more open to sharing her feelings and trusts others more.

Indeed, de-emphasizing the role of food in relationships with food buddies can actually help friends change for the better, as Katie G. points out. "For a while," she says, "I didn't see a couple of friends. Our relationships had been based on conversations about our fat rolls while we pigged out on Peanut Buster Parfaits. We've advanced and have found more in common." Dorothy J. has shifted to new activities with some of her still-heavy friends: "We attend a play rather than eat together."

**The opposite sex may take notice.** Sandy P. finds it amusing that "after I initially lost weight 10 years ago, people who didn't talk to me before, especially men, took an interest." Liane F. notes that while women are jealous of her 29-pound loss, men give her more attention.

**Your friends may become healthier along with you.** Since losing her 65 pounds, Suzanne T. has "recruited" friends to join her exercise program and adds, "We share eating habits and encourage one another." Cathy B. comments, "Some of my old food buddies have discovered weight training or other interests that have better payoffs than eating."

WHAT DO YOU DO WHEN . . .

# You Want to Quit Smoking?

YOU'VE LOST THE WEIGHT AND FEEL SO GOOD that now you want to clean up your act even more by quitting smoking. Twenty-eight masters are living proof that it can be done, although it's not always easy. As Alicia G. states, "Quitting was hard—I screamed a lot, and I chewed on plastic straws." That was two years after she had mastered a 145-pound weight loss. She quit cold turkey. Alicia found it helpful to suck on sugar-free hard candies and drink a lot of Diet Coke. She recalls, "I almost always had to have something in my hand." She also wrote in a personal journal, recording her feelings.

Like Alicia, a number of other masters found that being physically active helped them survive the process without gaining weight. Joseph C. thinks he was able to quit smoking without regaining his 23 pounds because he increased his jogging. *(Because of the health risks of smoking, any smoker or former smoker should be certain to consult with his or her physician before exercising.)* A few other masters quit smoking by undergoing hypnosis. As a result, Shirley C. exults, "I haven't had a cigarette for over 14 years!"

After Jeff B. quit smoking four years ago, he regained 40 pounds. However, he's since lost 20 of that and is satisfied, because he currently weighs 65 pounds less than his all-time high.

# IS WEIGHT GAIN INEVITABLE WHEN YOU KICK THE HABIT?

IT IS TRUE THAT WHEN PEOPLE QUIT SMOKING, they tend to gain weight—typically between 8 and 14 pounds. (Of course, that relatively small amount is far less risky than continuing to smoke.) According to Robert Klesges, Ph.D., of the University of Memphis, cigarette smoking does not help people *lose* weight—rather, in smokers, it seems to *prevent* the slow weight gain that occurs in most of us as we age. He emphasizes, "When smokers quit smoking, they merely return to the weight they would have been had they never smoked." Why do people tend to gain when they kick the habit? In part, because of a change in metabolism. Smoking appears to increase metabolic rate, at least for a short time after having a cigarette. Dr. Klesges also believes that people tend to increase their intake of fat and sugar after they quit, at least for a while.

A recent study, published in the *American Journal of Public Health*, supports Dr. Klesges' belief that weight gain after quitting smoking is associated with more than metabolic changes—at least for some people. Researchers who studied more than 2,000 men who had quit smoking found that although the average weight gain was about 8 pounds, 282 men were classified as "super-gainers," having put on at least 25 pounds. They ate more candy and increased their intake of hard liquor by nearly double the amount of men who didn't gain weight after quitting smoking. Moreover, since the super-gainers were less likely to have exercised strenuously *before* they quit smoking, the researchers suggest that they probably expended less energy after they stopped smoking. Not only does exercise seem to be helpful in preventing weight gain when you swear off cigarettes, but there is also evidence that by increasing activity levels, the success rate of quitting smoking also increases.

Only a few masters quit smoking and lost weight at the same time. Weight-control expert John Foreyt, Ph.D., coauthor of *The New Living Heart Diet,* states that it's wise not to tackle both at once. Most experts emphasize quitting smoking *first,* because it's a more serious problem than being moderately overweight. The majority of masters who quit smoking quit *before* they lost their weight. For Randy W., quitting became the impetus for his 55-pound weight loss of 18 years ago. "When I quit smoking," he says, "I started walking as a substitute for cigarettes, and I actually lost some weight. I felt better and started exercising more." Eventually, his eating habits became more healthful.

Whether you want to quit smoking before or after you lose weight, healthy behaviors seem to come in packages—when people lick one detrimental habit, they commonly want to tackle others that are interfering with optimal health. Keith Van Gasken, director of Smoking Cessation for Health Management Resources in Boston, gained and then lost weight after quitting. He speaks from experience: "The more one engages in healthy lifestyle behaviors, the less likely it is that one will engage in unhealthy behaviors, like smoking."

WHAT DO YOU DO WHEN . . .
# You Find Out You're Pregnant?

PLANNED OR UNPLANNED PREGNANCIES can be unsettling for a once-heavy person, who must face the prospect of gaining 25 to 35 pounds, which is now the recommended amount for a healthy pregnancy in normal-weight women. Valerie D. explains, "I reached my goal and had my weight off for 3 months when I found out I was pregnant with my second child. I was devastated—I wanted to enjoy my weight loss for at least a year." She talked with her doctor, who had watched her lose the weight, and he encouraged her not to gain it back. She continued to go to her TOPS group, which offers special guidelines for pregnant members. "The first several months, I lost weight. My doctor had to get across to me that it was okay to gain."

All told, Valerie gained about 30 pounds and was back down to her prepregnancy weight within four months of having the baby. She advises, "Write down what you eat, be truthful and watch portions." Valerie, who didn't exercise when she was losing weight, also started walking when she was pregnant and continues to do so to keep her weight off.

Some masters got through pregnancy without gaining too much by focusing on eating healthfully, with the baby in mind. One of them, Debbie T., kept off her 62 pounds through two pregnancies, less than a year and a half apart. After the birth of her son, she states, "I was back down to my prepregnancy weight within six weeks." During pregnancy, she drank milk and ate yogurt and cheese. Her doctor suggested she try to control cravings, so Debbie would snack on popcorn and pretzels. When she occasionally craved chocolate, she would have a small bar. She also found it helpful to chew gum when she wanted to eat.

For Becky M., the first of five pregnancies—all of which occurred within 10 years—became the impetus for beginning a lifetime of healthful eating and exercising. She explains, "When I became pregnant, I stopped following goofy diets and decided to eat healthy. I also walked a lot. It wasn't just me and my appearance anymore—I wanted a healthy baby." Becky simply continued her new habits after giving birth and with each new pregnancy, never gaining more than 32 pounds. (She's been master of a 36-pound loss for 13 years, through all five pregnancies.)

Anna M., a 10-year master who gained 30 pounds during pregnancy, cut out sweets and ate "super-healthy—lots of fruits and vegetables, as well as yogurt and milk." From the seventh month on, she treated herself to a bowlful of ice cream each night, but she also exercised right up until she gave birth. She left the hospital just four pounds above her prepregnancy weight. Her troubles hit *after* she had the baby, while on her maternity leave, when she gained back 10 pounds. She nursed for five months, which increases calorie needs somewhat, but she snacked more and continued to eat ice cream regularly. To make matters worse, she found it difficult to exercise. When it was time to go back to work and her business clothes didn't fit, Anna went on a well-balanced diet, kept a food diary and got back down to 118 pounds, where she is today.

Cindy F., who had kept more than 100 pounds at bay for 9 years, dropped 20 of the 40 pounds she gained during pregnancy soon after she had her baby but gradually began to gain again. "So much energy was spent on the baby that I couldn't make weight control a priority. It was hard to find time to go to a Weight Watchers class, I didn't keep track of what I ate, and it was easier to grab fast food than to cut up carrot sticks or cook Weight Watchers recipes. I was also in the mode of eating more during pregnancy, and that was hard to break." After her daughter's first birthday, Cindy watched videotapes of herself and decided, "I'm not going back up to 285 pounds." She mustered the courage to return to Weight Watchers, weighing in at 210 pounds. "I had been a major Weight Watchers success story. In the past, I was a spokesperson for them, so it was hard to go back. But I found the support I need and found others in the same situation." Cindy is now on her way back down to her weight goal of 160, which is realistic, given her history and her height, which is 5'8".

The masters' message: *Eat healthfully, keeping the baby's needs in mind, keep track of what you eat, control your cravings, and with your physician's permission, get some exercise.*

WHAT DO YOU DO WHEN . . .

# Tragedy Strikes?

LESS THAN A YEAR AGO, when Ann F. was 43, her husband of eight years died suddenly. "It's really easy to go back and turn to food during depression," she says. "There are times when I feel, 'Who cares?'" But 11 years of maintaining a weight loss of more than 200 pounds has taught Ann that although turning to food may lift her spirits temporarily, "overeating really does feel terrible to me now." When she wants to comfort herself with food, Ann tries to reason herself out of it. "Sometimes it works; sometimes it doesn't." But when she slips, she forgives herself: "I'm not punitive, or it gets worse."

Her advice to others is, "Try to figure out what's really going to soothe you. Take a bath, stay in bed all day, go away for the weekend."

Ann feels it has helped her to make a special effort to eat a healthful, well-balanced diet. And she buys herself treats like "really good coffee." She also finds solace in her hobby of poetry writing. She joined a gym and finds that exercise helps as well.

Randy W. turned to exercise when he lost a loved one. Several years ago, his wife died of cancer. At the time, he says, "I lost more weight and exercised more. When other things in my life were out of control, working out longer and harder gave me a sense of control."

Terri M., too, finds that maintaining her 75-pound loss is a way of exerting control in the midst of sorrow. When her 23-year-old son drowned a year and a half ago, she says, "I wanted to give up." She credits her survival through the tragedy to her "TOPS family," whom she didn't want to disappoint by regaining. She feels it is critical to have a "genuine support network" when dealing with grief. Terri also continues to keep her weight off because of her late son. "He was so proud of me," she recalls; "I don't want to let him down to this day." If tragedy strikes, she advises, "if you need to grieve, grieve. Don't hide it, or it will come out in ways like overeating. There's a lot that's going to happen in life that you can't control, but you *can* control your weight."

WHAT DO YOU DO WHEN . . .

# You Eat No Fat, They Eat No Lean?

WHAT DO YOU DO WHEN YOUR EATING HABITS are different from those of the people with whom you live? About half the masters say they eat differently from the rest of their families or spouses. Some live with people who are overweight but make no effort to change their eating habits. Others have family members who don't really need to watch their weight. The masters who eat differently from their families seem to take things in stride. They offer the following solutions for dealing with those you live with:

**Eat something different.** About 20 masters indicated that at least some of the time, they eat different food from their families or spouses at mealtime. For Peppi S. and her husband, the solution is clear-cut: "I fix my meals, my husband fixes his meals." Virginia L. states, "My husband can eat anything he wants—usually fat, sweet, creamy. But I have my own side of the fridge with my allowable kinds of food. Sometimes, he likes my 'goodies' better!" Some masters cook low-fat versions of what they're serving the family for themselves. For instance, Shirley C. might make herself fat-free hot dogs when she cooks higher-fat foods for others at a family barbecue.

**Eat less of what they eat.** Quite a few masters eat what their families eat, but in smaller quantities. Joy C. explains, "Probably 50 percent of the time, I eat what my family eats, but small amounts of the high-fat foods. I add a big tossed salad or cabbage salad four to five nights a week—plus a vegetable and a starch like potatoes or rice."

**Avoid certain of their foods.** Some masters just view certain foods as "theirs, not mine." For instance, Carolyn S., whose husband "is not interested in dieting," notes, "I pass by a lot of things he eats." When her son lived at home, Lynne C. asked him to keep "treats" in his room. Joanna M. has a good solution: "I try to buy food that I'm not wild about for the children."

*Quite a few of the masters report that they've won their families over to more healthful eating.* Eileen K. declares, "I have just told my family that this is the way I cook now, and we are eating this way. If they want something else, then they can make their own." During most of the 15 years that Dorothy J. has been master of a 40-pound loss, her husband continued to eat a very high-fat diet. However, just recently, at 56, he went to his physician for fatigue and rapid heartbeat and wound up having quadruple-bypass heart surgery. His doctor admonished, "You need to make a complete lifestyle change—immediately!" As a result, Dorothy says, "We now have the chance to live a healthy, 'thin for life' way as we eat right and exercise together."

# You Want to Eat Out?

A T FIRST, IT CAN BE UNSETTLING to be faced with menu choices and the uncertainty of how food is prepared. But the masters don't let these factors scare them away: 7 out of 10 dine in restaurants *at least* once or twice a week. That's a lot more frequently than I would have guessed, since people often complain about how difficult it is to eat out and watch their weight.

Joanne F. learned to avoid restaurants where there were no good choices. She explains that in places that lack healthful choices, "it's too hard for me to eat a little bit. Now, if someone asks me where I'd like to go, I never say, 'Wherever you want.' *I* pick because I don't want to be set up to overeat." Joanne favors steak houses, which may seem odd for a vegetarian, but she finds that they're safe bets, because they always offer baked potatoes, salads and often steamed vegetables. (She tries not to go too often to Mexican restaurants, because she adores their nachos and other high-fat fare.) If Joanne isn't able to choose the restaurant, she tries to find out in advance what type of food it serves so she can plan what she'll have or figure out whether to bring some of her own food along, like nonfat butter spray or her own low-fat salad dressing.

When she's dining out, her guiding principle is, "Don't be afraid to ask for what you want. You are the customer!" She suggests, "Ask for broiled fish, no sauce or butter on the veggies, dressing on the side. Ask for things even if they're not on the menu. Most people are happy to accommodate." Knowing that restaurants often serve huge portions, Joanne sometimes does what a number of other masters do: she asks for a "to-go" container when she orders. Then, before she starts eating, she puts half the food in the container and moves it out of sight. To fill up, she also drinks a few glasses of water before her food arrives.

Many masters avoid fast-food restaurants entirely. Bret R. speaks for scores of masters when he says, "I almost never eat at fast-food restaurants—it's the kiss of death or, rather, fat."

# 10 Tips for Dining in Restaurants— Without Gaining Back Your Weight

**1. Be choosy about restaurants.** Liane F. says it succinctly, "I go to restaurants where I can have a low-fat meal—for example, pastas with red sauces and salads." Rita B. adds, "If there isn't anything on the menu that I can eat, I leave."

**2. Avoid buffets.** Even though low-fat choices might be available at all-you-can-eat-type restaurants, many masters stay away from them. Teresa M. explains why: "If a buffet is involved, then I'll always overeat." Patsy K. adds, "I cannot resist all the temptation: I always want to make sure I get my money's worth."

**3. Order wisely.** The healthful choices *are* usually there, perhaps buried in a list of foods like Reuben sandwiches, fried chicken and beef stroganoff. Accordingly, Jacque M. explains, "I read the menu carefully for the kinds of foods and how they are prepared. I try and order from a 'lite' or 'healthy' menu list." Similarly, Wendy M. says she orders "healthy-heart meals, a salad and fruit for dessert." (Be aware, however, that a recent Center for Science in the Public Interest analysis of "lite" and "healthy" entrées from seven large restaurant chains revealed that these special offerings are often higher in fat than the menus say.) Tybie K. offers another great tip for placing an order: "I make my choices quickly and try not to be influenced by others."

**4. Be assertive.** Making inquiries and giving special directions in restaurants are both important, because additions like butter and mayonnaise can crop up in the most unlikely places. Lynne C.'s policy is, "I ask a lot of questions and give directions quite clearly but not obnoxiously."

**5. Have it cooked right.** Just as when they eat at home, the masters specify low-fat cooking methods when they dine out. For Marie C., it's "broiled, baked or grilled dishes." Shirley C.'s approach is, "I look the waitperson straight in the eyes, smile with determination and say, 'I'm allergic to butter, so please have the chef prepare my vegetables by steaming and omit ALL sauces.'"

**6. Hold the fatty condiments.** Since small amounts of high-fat extras—like butter, margarine, salad dressings and sour cream—can quickly add up, the masters go out of their way to avoid them in restaurants. Chuck B. eats his rolls and bread plain. He reports, "I don't use the butter, and I ask for dressing on the side."

**7. Fill up on vegetables.** Many masters rely on salads when they eat at restaurants. Mabel H. explains, "I order a nice salad with lots of vegetables and a small amount of chicken, and that fills me up."

**8. Order "white" meat.** The masters tend to make the same protein choices in restaurants as they do at home. Chuck B. stresses, "I order fish or chicken as opposed to red meats." Tami B. orders fish or seafood, because the portions are small.

**9. Control portions.** Restaurant portions are often huge, so some masters go out of their way to order small portions. Dorothy C. might order two appetizers, which tend to be smaller than entrées, or an appetizer and a salad. Sharing food helps many masters too. Rose B. often buys one dinner and shares it with a friend, and they order two salads. Lynda M. takes a more unusual approach to limit what she eats: "Before I take the first bite, I separate out the amount I plan to eat and then I douse the rest with pepper or salt to make it inedible."

**10. Make allowances.** Whether they splurge a little or save up for restaurant meals during the day, some masters make special allowances when they dine out. Linda W., who usually goes out of her way to make low-fat choices in restaurants, makes the following exception: "If fettuccine Alfredo is offered, I will probably order it, enjoy it and not do that again for at least several weeks."

Others do their homework and seek out low-fat options (see "Saving Calories and Fat in Restaurants," page 102). Dolores M.H. says, "I read their brochures to find out which foods are lower in calories and fat." (If you eat in fast-food restaurants regularly, you should periodically restudy their nutrition information, since fast-food companies routinely tinker with recipes, according to the consumer group Center for Science in the Public Interest.)

A number of masters simply eat small portions of higher-fat items when frequenting fast-food spots. Charlotte M. advises, "If you want a hamburger and fries, pick a regular small burger and small fries." Thalia A.'s solution: "I have a standard McDonald's order of one small plain hamburger, a side garden salad (only lemon on the salad) and a glass of water. By the time I've eaten the salad, the small hamburger is enough for a 'burger' experience."

Finally, the masters have found that it never hurts to make special requests when ordering fast and take-out foods. At fast-food Mexican restaurants, Joanne F. specifies, "No cheese, no sour cream. I turn their seven-layer burrito into a three-layer one." She is also one of several masters who order vegetarian pizza—it's got the crust, sauce and extra vegetables, but no cheese or meat. Others request minimal oil when they order Chinese food. (See the chart on page 102 for specific lower-fat Chinese-food ideas.)

# Saving Calories and Fat in Restaurants*

| INSTEAD OF: | CHOOSE: | YOU WILL SAVE: Calories | Fat (grams) |
|---|---|---|---|
| **Fast Food** | | | |
| Burger King Double Whopper with Cheese | Burger King Cheeseburger with a Side Salad/Reduced-Calorie Dressing | 505 | 40 |
| KFC Original Recipe Chicken Breast | KFC Tender Roast Chicken Breast (skin removed) | 231 | 20 |
| Wendy's Biggie French Fries | Wendy's Baked Potato with Sour Cream & Chives | 80 | 17 |
| | with Barbecue Sauce | 100 | 23 |
| Arby's Chicken Breast Fillet (breaded) Sandwich | Arby's Light Roast Beef Deluxe Sandwich | 240 | 18 |
| McDonald's Filet-O-Fish Sandwich | McDonald's McGrilled Chicken Classic Sandwich (without sauce) | 100 | 12 |
| **Chinese** | | | |
| 1 Egg Roll | 1 cup Egg Drop Soup | 147 | 10 |
| 1 cup Fried Rice | 1 cup Steamed Rice | 59 | 14 |
| 8 ounces Mu Shu Chicken | 8 ounces Chicken with Snow Peas | 281 | 26 |
| 8 ounces Sweet and Sour Shrimp | 8 ounces Szechuan Shrimp | 243 | 12 |

| INSTEAD OF: | CHOOSE: | YOU WILL SAVE: Calories | Fat (grams) |
|---|---|---|---|
| **Mexican** | | | |
| 2 Burritos | 2 Chicken Fajitas | 94 | 5 |
| Taco Salad in Tortilla Shell with ground beef, cheese, salsa, tomato, lettuce, guacamole, sour cream | Taco Salad with a Flour Tortilla (no shell) with ground beef, cheese, extra salsa, tomato, lettuce | 151 | 18 |
| Deluxe Nachos: chips, beef, cheese, sour cream | 2 ounces tortilla chips with ½ cup salsa | 414 | 33 |
| **Italian** | | | |
| One-fourth 12-inch Pepperoni Deep-Dish Pizza | One-fourth 12-inch Thin Crust Pizza with vegetables | 245 | 14 |
| 4 ounces Fried Calamari | 1 cup Minestrone Soup | 93 | 6 |
| 1 cup Caesar Salad with Croutons | 1 cup Tossed Salad with Fat-Free Dressing | 137 | 12 |
| 16 ounces Lasagna | 16 ounces Linguine with Red Clam Sauce | 103 | 11 |
| 16 ounces Fettuccine Alfredo | 16 ounces Spaghetti with Tomato Sauce | 426 | 29 |

| INSTEAD OF: | CHOOSE: | YOU WILL SAVE: | |
| | | Calories | Fat (grams) |
| --- | --- | --- | --- |
| 1 slice Buttered Garlic Bread | 1 slice Plain Italian Bread | 28 | 4 |

**All-American**

| INSTEAD OF: | CHOOSE: | Calories | Fat |
| --- | --- | --- | --- |
| 10 ounces Prime Rib of Beef, fat trimmed | 8 ounces Filet Mignon | 335 | 23 |
| Grilled Cheese Sandwich | 3 ounces Smoked Turkey Breast on Rye with Mustard | 218 | 24 |
| ½ cup Coleslaw | ½ cup Steamed Carrots | 68 | 7 |
| 6 Deep-Fried Mushrooms | Shrimp Cocktail (6 shrimp plus shrimp sauce) | 59 | 12 |
| 6 ounces Fillet of Sole in White Cream Sauce | 6 ounces Broiled Haddock Fillet | 185 | 14 |
| Cherry Pie à la Mode (⅛ pie, ½ cup ice cream) | Cherries Jubilee (½ cup) with Whipped Topping | 408 | 27 |
| Hot Fudge Sundae (1 cup ice cream, ¼ cup hot fudge, ¼ cup whipped cream) | Frozen Yogurt (1 cup) | 458 | 34 |

*\* Restaurants vary; some use more fat than others. All nutrition values are subject to change. This information was accurate as of August 1996.*

# You Go to Parties, Weddings and Dinners?

WHEN YOU ARE TRYING TO WATCH YOUR WEIGHT, parties, weddings and dining at friends' homes can pose more of a challenge than eating in restaurants, because you typically have less control. As Shirley G. puts it, "Parties and weddings are very tough for me. I usually overeat—or shall I say eat like everyone else. Then I compensate either the day before or the day after." The masters have evolved various ways of taking a stand on social situations involving food:

◆ **Have small amounts of what's offered.** This is by far the most commonly mentioned method of handling social occasions. Marjorie C. remarks, "I take only very small portions—I skip the mints and nuts."

◆ **Station yourself away from food.** If you're standing right next to the chips, you're bound to eat them. Charlotte M. says, "I stay away from the hors d'oeuvres table."

◆ **Focus on activities other than eating.** Another way masters cope with social events is to mingle. Joanne F. says, "I socialize or get involved with things other than the food."

◆ **Seek out healthful choices.** Many masters make an effort to find the low-fat, low-calorie items now commonly available when people party. Susan M. states, "I snack on the vegetables."

◆ **Plan ahead.** A number of masters go out of their way to anticipate what will be served and plan accordingly. Thalia A. explains, "I visualize how I want to eat and what choices I'll make." A few people even call ahead to see what will be offered. Lynda C. says, "If I know the party-givers, I ask what's going to be there. If nothing is there that falls within my parameters of food, I'll either eat before I go or bring my own."

◆ **Fill up on no-calorie beverages.** "Request a glass of water with lemon while you mingle," Mary Ann K. recommends. Joanne F. points out, "If you keep a glass of seltzer or pop in your hand or in a wineglass, no one will ask to fill your drink."

◆ **Eat less at other times.** A number of masters consciously "save up" or "make up" for food eaten at social events, allowing themselves to splurge a little. Peppi S. states, "I usually try and eat whatever I want, within reason. I may eat less before and after the event to balance it out."

◆ **Choose the best.** Quite a few masters are selective and make sure they spend their calories the way they want to. Tami B.'s approach is, "At weddings, I skip the food and go for the cake; at parties, I pick and choose the best foods and enjoy."

As always, the masters usually combine several techniques when dealing with social events. For example, not only does JoAnna L. (130 pounds, 3 years) concentrate on visiting with people she hasn't seen in a while, but, "I look at everything that is offered before putting anything on my plate. I make the best decisions based on what there is, and I don't go back for seconds."

# You Go on Vacation?

SINCE VACATIONS CAN SIGNAL "FREE TIME"—not just schedule-wise but foodwise—I asked each master, "How do you handle your food intake when on vacation?" *The vast majority said they make an effort to do the same things they do at home to control their weight.* In other words, many of them try to follow their low-fat eating habits and continue to exercise when they vacation. Tim H.'s guiding philosophy is, "I realize that I am on vacation but will be returning with the same body. There's no free lunch!"

Joanne F. goes one step further and keeps a food diary, something she does only occasionally at home. She remarks, "Going back to some of my more stringent habits helps me keep my head." Many other masters make an effort to take along low-fat foods and snacks. Irene H. explains, "I carry special food in a cooler and watch where we eat so I can order the right foods. In the past two years, every time we have gone on vacation, I have lost up to 3 pounds."

*None of this is to say that the masters don't treat themselves while vacationing.* Ann F. says, "I like to snack and visit candy stores, so I try to have fruit for breakfast and salad at one meal." Peppi S. tries to eat pasta or chicken, vegetables and fruits for at least one meal, so she "can enjoy the luxury of a treat or higher-calorie food once or twice on the trip."

Other masters splurge with more abandon and pay the consequences later. Carlton R. is typical of these: "On vacation, I usually 'pig out,' knowing I can return to normal when I return home."

Another approach used by certain masters on vacation is best summed up by Patsy K., who advises, "Do fun things that aren't centered around food." *In other words, keep busy.* Charlotte M. urges, "Indulge, enjoy and walk yourself crazy!"

The masters have found ways to cope with life's challenges without gaining back their weight. As Joanne says, "When I face challenges and I want to eat, I realize I'm still going to have the problems afterward. Now, I can look at my 'before' photo on the bathroom wall and know that the effort is all worthwhile."

# PART II

# MEALS
## *from the*
# MASTERS

## CHAPTER SIX

Meals from the Masters:

# The Ultimate Low-Fat, Low-Calorie 21-Day Weight-Loss Plan

T O DIET OR NOT TO DIET? It almost goes without saying that to lose weight, you have to eat less than you're currently eating. So do you go on some sort of a diet or structured food plan *or* do you follow a nondieting approach—simply cutting back and trying to eat more healthful foods? (About half of the masters I spoke with for *Thin for Life* lost weight on their own; the other half sought assistance to slim down.) How do you know which method is best for you?

It helps to look at your past attempts, examining what did and didn't work for you. If you did well on a weight-loss program with a specific food plan plus group and/or professional support, you should consider going back. (See it as a sign of strength, not failure, that you are willing to seek help for your weight problem once again.) If you choose this route, it's important that the plan be tailored to your individual needs and preferences so that from the outset, you're beginning to forge habits you can stick with for a lifetime. (If you are selecting a weight-loss program for the first time, be sure to shop around and ask a lot of questions.)

*The masters make it clear that there is no one solution that applies to all individuals.* In fact, I have a strong hunch that one reason so many people fail with popular weight-loss approaches is that they latch on to trendy diet books based on a single individual's experience, one the author espouses as "the way" to successful weight control. In so doing, would-be weight losers fail to find what's right for them. But the masters' examples show us that within some basic parameters, there are many ways to lick the problem.

*Many masters did use diets to get their weight off.* (Most who dieted sought help from weight-loss organizations rather than doing it on their own.) As long as you truly accept the need to change your habits permanently, diets can be useful tools to launch you on your way to a new food life.

*On the other hand, if you've had it with diets and with other people giving you advice on how to lose weight, a nondieting approach may be for you.* Masters who lost weight on their own typically used a self-styled approach, changing their lifestyles gradually, focusing on healthful eating, watching fat and calories, and increasing exercise.

In part, whether or not you diet depends on how patient you are and how much you weigh. Slow weight loss may be particularly difficult to stick with if you have a lot to lose—say, 50 pounds or more; some heavy people do better with a more aggressive, medically supervised approach.

*If you want to lose weight on your own but you're not a "program" person, and if you've done well on low-calorie diets in the past, a sensible fat- and calorie-restricted food plan, such as Meals from the Masters, may be right for you.*

# Meals from the Masters

I F YOU'RE LIKE MANY VETERAN DIETERS, it often feels overwhelming to put together low-fat foods in reasonable amounts in a variety of satisfying meals. Meals from the Masters, based on the masters' favorites, is a weight-loss plan to get you started—and one you can build on and gradually expand when you get to maintenance. It gives you 21 days' worth of ideas so you can lose weight without boredom. Soon, you'll get the hang of planning low-fat meals with daily treats on your own.

A day's worth of meals (excluding snacks) averages around 1,170 calories. To lose weight safely on your own, women should go no lower than 1,200 calories per day, so they should be sure to include one snack each day in addition to their three meals. Men who are shedding pounds on their own should consume no fewer than 1,500 calories and thus should increase the portion sizes given here somewhat. (For instance, to add another 300 calories to any single day's food plan, men could add another cup of skim milk, a slice of bread, a large piece of fruit and a pat of margarine.) Most women can expect to lose 1 to 2 pounds a week on this plan, depending on individual calorie needs and the amount of exercise they do; men may lose more.

All the meals included here are easy to prepare and require no fancy recipes. Each breakfast provides no more than 300 calories; lunches have 400 calories or less; suppers have no more than 500 calories. *You should be certain to eat three daily meals from the plan, along with a snack from either of the two snack lists*—one with 100-calorie items, the other with 200-calorie snacks. With Meals from the Masters, you need not worry about counting fat grams, because the proportion of calories from fat for the entire plan comes out to less than 20 percent, which is surprisingly low for all the delicious foods you get to eat.

Some meals include additions of foods like butter, regular salad dressing or maple syrup—as opposed to nonfat or low-calorie versions. It's fine if you choose to use low-fat/low-calorie versions of these items and spend the saved calories elsewhere, say by increasing the portion size of another food (such as pasta) a bit. Conversely, since the meals do tend to be so low in fat, you may substitute some low-fat or reduced-fat items for nonfat versions—as long as product labels indicate that calorie levels are similar. Occasionally, you may substitute similar foods for any one food on a meal plan. For example, if you dislike asparagus, you can substitute another green vegetable, such as broccoli. Or you could substitute a "light" beer for a glass of wine or use canned salmon in place of steamed. (It's wise to consult product labels or a calorie/fat reference book to make sure calorie and fat levels of the two items are similar.)

It is important to include a wide variety of meals from each of the categories in order to assure nutritional adequacy. (See guidelines for the recommended number of servings from each food group, on pages 56 to 57.) Calcium and iron are two nutrients likely to be in short supply when women, in particular, are trying to lose weight. Ideally, you should have at least three good sources of calcium* each day, as well as one vitamin-C-rich food (citrus fruits and juices, strawberries, cantaloupe, honeydew melon, broccoli, cauliflower, Brussels sprouts, green peppers, tomatoes, cabbage, spinach and asparagus) and one good source of beta carotene/vitamin A (carrots, pumpkin, sweet potatoes, spinach, winter squash, dark greens, apricots, broccoli and watermelon).

When following this or any low-calorie food plan for more than a week or two, it is wise to take a multivitamin/mineral supplement containing 100 percent of the recommended daily amount for vitamins and minerals (marked "100% Daily Value" on the label). This will also help women meet their iron needs. In keeping with the masters' advice (and with good health practices), be sure to drink at least six to eight 8-ounce cups of water or noncaffeinated liquids each day.

*As with any weight-reduction plan, it is advised that you first get your physician's approval before following Meals from the Masters.* If you have any medical problems or if you have more than 20 pounds to lose, you should be monitored by your physician as you are losing weight. If you feel weak or experience any adverse physical changes while following Meals from the Masters, consult your physician. These food plans are not designed for pregnant or nursing women,

---

\* *The National Institutes of Health's recommendation for daily calcium intake for adults ages 25 to 64 is 1,000 milligrams for men, premenopausal women and postmenopausal women who take estrogen; 1,500 milligrams of calcium is recommended for postmenopausal women who are not taking estrogen. Men and women over the age of 65 should consume 1,500 milligrams a day.*

*The following foods provide about 300 milligrams of calcium: 1 cup skim or low-fat milk, ½ cup evaporated skim milk, 1 cup buttermilk, 8 ounces yogurt, 1½ ounces reduced-fat cheese, 1 cup calcium-fortified juice, 4 ounces salmon or mackerel (canned, with bones). Foods that provide approximately 150 milligrams of calcium include: 1 cup broccoli, ½ cup pudding or custard, ¾ cup ice milk or ice cream, ¾ cup frozen yogurt, 1 cup cottage cheese. If you don't consume enough of these foods or if you want to find out whether you're getting enough calcium, you should check with your physician and a registered dietitian who can advise whether you should take a calcium supplement.*

children or teenagers or for people with medical problems. People who are on a special diet, such as low-sodium, should check with a dietitian and physician before following Meals from the Masters.

**Notes About Specific Foods in Meals from the Masters:**
♦ Reduced-fat cheeses should have no more than 5 grams of fat per ounce.
♦ Reduced-calorie salad dressings should have no more than 40 calories per tablespoon.
♦ Eggs are assumed to be large.
♦ In the nutrition analyses, "negligible fat" means that a particular meal plan has less than 1 gram of fat.

# 21 Eye-Opener Breakfasts from the Masters

### (300 calories or less)

♦ Cream of Wheat: 3 tablespoons dry Cream of Wheat, 8 ounces skim milk, 1 tablespoon chopped dates
4 ounces orange juice

| Calories: 292 | Fat: negligible | (Paul A.) |

♦ 1 mug hot cocoa (made with 8 ounces skim milk, 1 tablespoon cocoa powder and low-calorie sweetener to taste)
2 slices whole wheat toast, each with 1 teaspoon reduced-fat margarine

| Calories: 292 | Fat: 7.5 grams | (Rose B.) |

- 1 slice whole wheat toast with 1 tablespoon reduced-fat peanut butter
  8 ounces skim milk with 1 teaspoon almond extract and 1 packet
  low-calorie sweetener
      Calories: 274        Fat: 7.5 grams        (Jennifer B.)

> "When you're not hungry, go survey the grocery store
> and notice all the foods out there that are lower in
> fat—there are many!" —Jennifer B.

- 1 poached egg sprinkled with 1 teaspoon bacon bits
  1 slice whole wheat toast with 1 tablespoon raspberry jam
  6 ounces grapefruit juice
      Calories: 294        Fat: 7 grams        (Joy C.)

- 3-Variety Cereal: 1 Shredded Wheat bar, 2 tablespoons Grape-
  Nuts, ¼ cup puffed rice
  Top with ½ medium banana (sliced)
  8 ounces skim milk
      Calories: 284        Fat: 1 gram        (Shirley C.)

- Reduced-fat bran muffin (2-ounce)
  ½ cup grapes
  6 ounces orange juice
      Calories: 297        Fat: 5.5 grams        (Marie C.)

> "Every moment is a new start; you don't have to wait
> until Monday to get healthier." —Kathy B.

- 1 blueberry bagel (2½-ounce) with 2 teaspoons nonfat cream
  cheese
  Skinny Latte: 8 ounces strong coffee with 8 ounces steamed skim milk
      Calories: 300        Fat: 2.5 grams        (Judy C.)

* French Toast: 2 slices reduced-calorie whole wheat bread, ¼ cup egg substitute, 1 teaspoon vanilla extract, 1 packet low-calorie sweetener, 2 tablespoons skim milk (cook in a nonstick skillet sprayed with nonstick butter-flavored spray); top with 2 table-spoons reduced-calorie pancake syrup
1 slice honeydew melon

  Calories: 286          Fat: 3.5 grams          (David D.)

* Yogurt "Sundae": Layer in a brandy snifter: ¼ cup fresh blue-berries, ½ sliced peach, ¼ cup sliced strawberries, 4 ounces raspberry yogurt (nonfat, sweetened with aspartame); repeat; top with 3 tablespoons reduced-fat granola

  Calories: 286          Fat: 2 grams          (Ann F.)

> "Try not to get too hungry. Give your body enough
> nourishing and tasty food, and you won't be as
> driven to overeat." —Ann F.

* ½ cup cooked oatmeal (made with skim milk) mixed with ½ cup nonfat sugar-free vanilla pudding
1 slice reduced-calorie toast with 1 teaspoon reduced-fat peanut butter and 1 teaspoon honey

  Calories: 281          Fat: 4 grams          (Cindy F.)

* Breakfast Shake: 6 ounces strawberry yogurt (nonfat, sweetened with aspartame), 1 medium banana, 1 tablespoon wheat germ, ⅓ cup skim milk, ¼ cup orange juice (blend all ingredients in a blender until smooth)

  Calories: 270          Fat: 1.5 grams          (Katie G.)

* Veggie Scramble: Microwave or steam 1 cup mixed vegetables (chopped broccoli, onion, green pepper, mushrooms); scramble

with 1 whole egg, 1 egg white, ¼ cup skim milk and 1 slice
(¾-ounce) crumbled low-fat cheese in a nonstick skillet
6 ounces orange juice

Calories: 295          Fat: 9.5 grams                    (Joe K.)


♦ 2 slices cinnamon-raisin toast, each spread with 2 tablespoons
warm applesauce (unsweetened), sprinkled with cinnamon
8 ounces skim milk

Calories: 294          Fat: 4.5 grams                    (Nancy K. )


♦ "Jo's Granola": ¾ cup corn flakes, 1 tablespoon raisins, 1 small
banana (sliced), 2 teaspoons chopped pecans, brown-sugar
substitute
8 ounces skim milk

Calories: 292          Fat: 4.5 grams                    (JoAnna L.)


♦ ⅓ cup uncooked oatmeal prepared with 8 ounces skim milk; top
with ½ tablespoon strawberry or raspberry jam
6 ounces freshly squeezed orange juice

Calories: 297          Fat: 2.5 grams                    (Dean M.)


♦ ½ medium cantaloupe
1 egg scrambled with ¼ cup sliced mushrooms, plus chives and
basil, topped with 3 tablespoons salsa
1 slice whole wheat toast with 2 teaspoons apricot preserves

Calories: 300          Fat: 7.5 grams                    (Lynda M.)


♦ 2 low-fat buttermilk pancakes, topped with 2 teaspoons nonfat
margarine and 2 tablespoons real maple syrup
½ small pear, sliced

Calories: 300          Fat: 4 grams                    (Don Mauer)

♦ 2 fat-free waffles, topped with 1 teaspoon real butter and
   2 tablespoons reduced-calorie pancake syrup
   ½ grapefruit

   Calories: 296          Fat: 4 grams          (Cindy P.)

> "I dip my pancake or waffle into the syrup
> instead of pouring it on. That way,
> I don't use as much." —Cindy P.

♦ 1 toasted oat-bran waffle, topped with ⅓ cup nonfat cottage
   cheese
   Drizzle with 2 teaspoons honey and sprinkle with nutmeg
   6 ounces orange juice

   Calories: 290          Fat: 4 grams          (Ann Q.)

♦ Toasted English muffin with 2 slices (¾ ounce each) nonfat cheese
   melted on top and sprinkled with seasoned pepper
   6 ounces orange juice

   Calories: 272          Fat: 1 gram          (Dorothy S.)

♦ ½ cup nonfat cottage cheese on a bed of fruit—1 peach half,
   10 red grapes, ½ medium pear, ½ cup sliced strawberries
   1 slice whole wheat cinnamon-raisin toast with 1 teaspoon nonfat
   margarine

   Calories: 295          Fat: 2.5 grams          (Bob W.)

> "I always take 'quiet time' every day—to pray and
> meditate with breakfast." —Bob W.

# 21 Light and Luscious Lunches from the Masters

## (400 calories or less)

- 1 medium baked potato, cut into chunks; serve on a bed of 2 cups tossed salad, topped with 3 tablespoons fat-free Catalina dressing
  6 ounces strawberry yogurt (nonfat, sweetened with aspartame)
  1 medium orange

  Calories: 398     Fat: 1 gram          (Patsy B.)

- 1 cup homemade bean soup with 1 ounce low-fat sausage
  1 slice whole-grain bread
  2 clementines (or tangerines)
  2 gingersnaps

  Calories: 391     Fat: 7.5 grams       (Jane Brody)

> "Gradually improve your diet by changing one meal
> a week to one that is low in fat and filled
> with health-promoting vegetables
> and fruits." —Jane Brody

- Cheese soufflé, made with 2 eggs and 2 ounces fat-free Cheddar cheese
  1 slice sourdough bread
  ¾ cup applesauce (no sugar added), sprinkled with cinnamon

  Calories: 378     Fat: 11 grams        (Jennie C.)

- Sandwich: 1 ounce lean corned beef on 2 slices low-calorie wheat bread, with 3 large leaves leaf lettuce and Dijon mustard

6 fat-free potato chips
1 fat-free fig bar
1 cup chocolate milk (8 ounces skim milk with 2 tablespoons
    chocolate syrup)
>    Calories: 384        Fat: 4.5 grams            (Shirley C.)

♦ Soft-Shelled Chicken Taco: 1 flour tortilla (8-inch), 2 ounces
    cooked chicken breast (in strips), ¼ cup salsa, ⅓ cup shredded
    lettuce, 1 ounce shredded reduced-fat Cheddar cheese,
    2 tablespoons nonfat sour cream
½ cup red grapes
>    Calories: 400        Fat: 10 grams             (Don C.)

♦ Chinese Chicken Salad: Gently toss 3 ounces cooked, cubed
    skinless chicken breast, 2 cups shredded cabbage, ½ sliced red
    or green pepper, ¼ cup sliced green onions, 1 teaspoon sugar,
    1 teaspoon sesame seeds, ½ tablespoon sesame oil; season to
    taste with salt or soy sauce, vinegar or lemon juice, pepper; top
    with ¼ cup chow mein noodles
¾ cup pineapple chunks (fresh or in juice)
>    Calories: 386        Fat: 15.5 grams           (Judy F.)

♦ Asparagus-Chicken Salad: 3 ounces cooked, boneless, skinless chicken
    breast (in strips), 1 medium tomato (sliced), 10 fresh asparagus
    spears (steamed); marinate in ¼ cup fat-free Italian dressing
6 reduced-fat wheat crackers
8 ounces peach yogurt (nonfat, sweetened with aspartame)
>    Calories: 390        Fat: 5.5 grams            (Ann F.)

> **"Plenty of low-fat dairy products and sweets taste good.
> Experiment—you won't stick with what you
> don't like." —Ann F.**

◆ Bagel Sandwich: 2 ounces shaved, smoked turkey breast on
   1 onion bagel with lettuce and 1 tablespoon nonfat mayonnaise
   1 large nectarine
   8 ounces skim milk

       Calories: 392      Fat: 3.5 grams      (Tom F.)

◆ From McDonald's restaurant: 1 chicken fajita; side salad with
   ½ packet barbecue sauce; chocolate low-fat frozen yogurt

       Calories: 382      Fat: 11 grams      (Julie J. )

      **"At fast-food restaurants, choose wisely. It's very doable,
      and you won't feel deprived." —Julie J.**

◆ Tuna-Pasta Salad: 2 ounces (drained) water-pack albacore tuna,
   1 cup cooked corkscrew pasta, 1 cup thawed frozen vegetables
   (broccoli, cauliflower, carrots, peas), 1 small chopped tomato,
   1 cup endive; toss with 1 tablespoon grated Parmesan cheese
   ½ cup raspberries (unsweetened)

       Calories: 399      Fat: 5 grams      (Patsy K.)

◆ "Jo's Power Sandwich": 2 slices reduced-calorie whole wheat bread,
   1 tablespoon plus 1 teaspoon reduced-fat peanut butter,
   1 tablespoon apple butter, ½ medium banana (sliced)
   8 ounces skim milk

       Calories: 388      Fat: 9.5 grams      (JoAnna L.)

◆ Vegetarian Sub: Italian roll (6-inch) with 1½ ounces shredded
   part-skim mozzarella, ¼ cup chopped green pepper, ½ medium
   tomato (sliced), ½ cup shredded lettuce, ½ small onion (sliced),
   2 tablespoons fat-free Italian dressing, 1 tablespoon mustard
   1 medium Granny Smith apple

       Calories: 396      Fat: 10 grams      (Don Mauer)

- Ham and Cheese on a Bun: 1 ounce extra-lean ham, 1 ounce
  fat-free Swiss cheese, 1 hamburger bun
  1 small can V-8
  ½ cup low-fat butterscotch pudding, topped with 2 tablespoons
  reduced-fat dessert topping
    Calories: 384    Fat: 6 grams    (Marlene R.)


- 1 cup tomato soup (such as Campbell's Healthy Request)
  Fat-Free Grilled Cheese Sandwich: 2 slices rye bread, 2 slices
    (1½ ounces) fat-free American cheese; grill in nonstick skillet
    coated with nonstick butter-flavored spray
  8 ounces skim milk (if desired, add 1 teaspoon vanilla and
    1 packet low-calorie sweetener)
    Calories: 379    Fat: 4 grams    (Emil R.)


- Whole wheat tortilla (8-inch) spread with 2 tablespoons fat-free
  "refried" beans and warmed; top with 2 tablespoons chopped
  onion, ½ medium tomato (sliced), 2 tablespoons salsa, ¼ cup
  shredded reduced-fat Cheddar cheese, 1 tablespoon nonfat
  sour cream
  3 slices fresh or canned juice-packed pineapple
    Calories: 391    Fat: 9 grams    (Bonnie R.)


- "Better-the-Second-Time" Salad made with leftover vegetables and
  cheese: for example, 2½ cups romaine lettuce; ½ cup each leftover
  cooked broccoli, cauliflower, sliced carrots; 1 ounce shredded
  regular Cheddar cheese; 2 tablespoons reduced-fat ranch dressing
  1 oatmeal cookie (2-inch)
    Calories: 372    Fat: 20.5 grams    (Leslie S.)

"Compared with when I was heavy, I eat much less—
except for salads. I often have salad as a
separate course." —Leslie S.

♦ 1 cup vegetarian vegetable soup
1 whole wheat bagel (2 ounces)
1 ounce string cheese (part-skim mozzarella)
20 Bing cherries

Calories: 397      Fat: 10 grams      (Kelly S.)

"I pack bagels, string cheese and fruit to take with me
when I'm out and about." —Kelly S.

♦ Pasta Salad: ¾ cup cooked rotini pasta, ¼ cup sliced fresh
mushrooms, ½ cup mixed vegetables (steamed), 2 tablespoons
fat-free Italian dressing
1-ounce breadstick
2 apricots
8 ounces skim milk

Calories: 374      Fat: 3 grams      (Debbie T.)

♦ Hearty Club Sandwich: 2 slices rye bread (toasted), 2 ounces
sliced smoked turkey breast, 1 thin slice (½ ounce) Swiss cheese,
½ medium tomato (sliced), 3 green pepper slices, 1 romaine
lettuce leaf, 4 cucumber slices, 1 tablespoon reduced-fat
mayonnaise
1 watermelon wedge (1-x-5-inch slice)

Calories: 373      Fat: 10.5 grams      (Carol W.)

♦ Open-Face Tuna Salad Sandwich: 2 slices whole wheat bread,
3 ounces water-packed tuna, 1½ tablespoons fat-free
mayonnaise, 2 teaspoons sweet-pickle relish
1 carrot cut into strips and dipped in 1 tablespoon fat-free ranch
dressing
1 large plum

Calories: 394          Fat: 4.5 grams          (Lorraine W.)

♦ Vegetarian Sandwich: 2 slices pumpernickel bread, ¼ cup each
shredded carrots and mung bean sprouts, 2 slices (1½ ounces)
fat-free American cheese, 2 teaspoons sunflower seeds,
1½ tablespoons fat-free mayonnaise
10 fat-free tortilla chips with ¼ cup salsa

Calories: 392          Fat: 6 grams          (Randy W.)

# 21 Satisfying Suppers from the Masters

## (500 calories or less)

♦ 1 cup fresh strawberries
3 ounces roasted turkey breast (skinless)
½ cup low-fat scalloped potatoes (made with skim milk and
reduced-calorie margarine)
½ cup fresh green beans, steamed
1 medium ear corn on the cob
Salad: 1 cup romaine lettuce, ⅓ cup cauliflower florets, 3 cherry
tomatoes, ½ sliced red pepper, ½ medium sliced carrot,
3 tablespoons fat-free blue cheese dressing

Calories: 499          Fat: 5.5 grams          (Rose B.)

"To fill up on nonfattening foods, I usually eat fresh
strawberries before dinner." —Rose B.

♦ Veggie Pizza: 10-inch pita bread, spread with ⅓ cup reduced-fat
   spaghetti or pizza sauce, topped with ¼ cup each onions, green
   peppers, broccoli, zucchini and mushrooms that have been stir-
   fried in a nonstick skillet; sprinkle with 1 tablespoon grated
   Parmesan cheese
¾ cup applesauce (no sugar added)
   Calories: 489      Fat: 4 grams            (Chuck B.)

♦ 4-ounce grilled rib-eye steak (weight after trimming and cooking)
   1 medium baked potato (4-ounce)
   1 tablespoon real sour cream with chives
   ½ cup steamed peas
   ⅙ medium cantaloupe
   Calories: 498      Fat: 17 grams           (Jean B.)

♦ Seafood Chef's Salad: 3 cups Boston lettuce, 3 ounces cooked fish
   (tuna, cod, halibut), ⅓ cup broccoli florets, 4 cherry tomatoes,
   1 medium carrot (shredded), 2 tablespoons vinaigrette dressing
   2 one-ounce slices warm French bread
   8 ounces skim milk
   Calories: 500      Fat: 9 grams            (Jane Brody)

♦ 1 grilled chicken breast (skinless, seasoned with saffron, if desired)
   1 cup spinach, steamed with 1 clove minced garlic and ½ medium
   chopped red pepper
   1½-ounce piece focaccia bread
   Greek Salad: 1 cup romaine lettuce, ½ ounce feta cheese,
   1 teaspoon olive oil, 2 teaspoons wine vinegar, 4 black olives
   Calories: 492      Fat: 16.5 grams         (Cathy B.)

"Buy a good low-fat cookbook and read magazines
with information and recipes for low-fat
but flavorful eating." —Marie C.


♦ 4 ounces grilled swordfish
1 medium baked potato (4-ounce) with 2 tablespoons fat-free
Peppercorn Ranch dressing
1 cup steamed spinach with ¼ cup diced tomatoes
1 cup shredded carrots with 1 tablespoon raisins, 2 tablespoons
fat-free French dressing and low-calorie sweetener to taste
  Calories: 485       Fat: 7.5 grams        (Pat C.)


♦ Eggplant Parmesan: 5 slices eggplant baked with ½ cup reduced-
fat spaghetti sauce and 1 ounce shredded part-skim
mozzarella cheese
½ cup cooked angel hair pasta
Salad with 1½ cups iceberg lettuce, ¼ cup bean sprouts,
½ cucumber, ½ medium tomato, 2 tablespoons reduced-calorie
Italian dressing
1-ounce breadstick
½ medium papaya
  Calories: 489       Fat: 8.5 grams        (Ann F.)


♦ 1¼ cups turkey chili (Hormel brand), topped with 2 tablespoons
nonfat sour cream and 1 ounce shredded reduced-fat Cheddar
cheese
10 baby carrots
5 unsalted saltines
  Calories: 496       Fat: 12.5 grams        (Julie J.)


♦ Southwestern Lasagna: 3 ounces cooked lasagna noodles (1½
noodles), layered with ½ cup nonfat cottage cheese, ⅓ cup salsa

and 1 ounce shredded reduced-fat Monterey Jack cheese
Garlic Breadstick: 1-ounce breadstick sprayed with butter-flavored
nonstick spray and sprinkled with garlic salt
1 cup steamed snap peas

Calories: 500     Fat: 9 grams     (Mary Ann K.)

"You didn't gain the weight overnight. Be patient—
it will come off when you are mentally ready to make a
healthy lifestyle change." —Mary Ann K.

◆ Joe's Simple Pasta and Vegetables: Microwave (all together) 1 small
sliced onion, ½ medium sliced green pepper and ⅓ cup each
broccoli florets, sliced carrots, zucchini slices and sliced
mushrooms; toss vegetables with 1 cup cooked spaghetti,
2 tablespoons reduced-calorie Italian dressing, 2 tablespoons
grated Parmesan cheese and garlic salt to taste
1-ounce slice French bread with 1 teaspoon margarine

Calories: 496     Fat: 13 grams     (Joe K. )

◆ 1 reduced-fat hot dog on a hot dog bun with 1 tablespoon
chopped onions
½ cup vegetarian baked beans
1 medium sliced tomato with basil, salt and pepper
8 ounces blueberry yogurt (nonfat, sweetened with aspartame)

Calories: 487     Fat: 11.5 grams     (Cam L.)

◆ 4 ounces grilled or broiled skinless chicken breast with
2 tablespoons barbecue sauce
1 cup steamed green beans, seasoned with liquid smoke
1 cup corn
1 medium baked potato, flavored with Molly McButter, salt and
pepper

Calories: 500     Fat: 5 grams     (Teresa M.)

- Linguine Tossed with Shrimp and Vegetables: 1 cup cooked
  linguine, 3 ounces steamed shrimp, ⅓ cup each steamed
  broccoli florets, mushrooms and carrot coins; 1 large clove
  garlic, minced and sautéed in 1 teaspoon olive oil; sprinkle with
  sweet basil and 1 tablespoon grated Parmesan cheese
  1½ cups romaine lettuce with ¼ cup sliced water chestnuts and
  2 tablespoons reduced-fat creamy Italian dressing
    Calories: 490      Fat: 13 grams            (Lynda M.)


- 4 ounces broiled Chilean sea bass
  2 cups salad, made with lettuce, red and green cabbage, red and
  green pepper, cucumber, carrots and dill pickle, with
  3 tablespoons reduced-fat blue cheese dressing
  2 large ears corn on the cob
    Calories: 491      Fat: 9.5 grams           (Diane S.)


- 4 ounces steamed salmon
  1 cup asparagus
  1 medium baked potato (4-ounce) with 1 pat butter
  Spinach Salad: 2 cups fresh spinach, 2 slices red onion, ⅓ cup
  sliced fresh mushrooms, 1 teaspoon bacon bits, 1 tablespoon
  honey-Dijon dressing
    Calories: 499      Fat: 17 grams            (Leslie S.)


- Large Salad: 2 cups leaf lettuce, ¼ cup each raw broccoli florets,
  sliced mushrooms, sliced celery and sliced green onions, with
  3 tablespoons fat-free Thousand Island dressing
  2 small chicken drumsticks, baked and skinned
  1 reduced-fat biscuit
  2 sliced kiwi fruits
  8 ounces skim milk
    Calories: 498      Fat: 7.5 grams           (Dorothy S.)

"At dinner, I start with a huge salad.
That leaves no room for oversized portions
of other foods." —Dorothy S.

♦ 4 ounces grilled teriyaki chicken breast
  1½ cups broccoli, with nutmeg and lemon juice
  6 small red-skin potatoes, roasted in 2 teaspoons olive oil and
    crushed garlic
  1 cup coleslaw, made with 1 cup shredded cabbage, 1 teaspoon
    sugar, 2 tablespoons nonfat mayonnaise and 2 teaspoons Dijon
    mustard
      Calories: 486      Fat: 14.5 grams      (Jim V.)

♦ Linguine with Stir-Fried Vegetables: 1 cup frozen stir-fry
    vegetables (steamed), 1½ ounces sliced low-fat sausage,
    served over a bed of 1 cup cooked linguine
  Caesar Salad: 1½ cups romaine lettuce, 10 green grapes, 1 ounce
    low-fat croutons (Italian bread cubes coated with nonstick spray
    and Italian seasoning, then toasted in oven), 2 tablespoons
    reduced-calorie Caesar dressing
      Calories: 499      Fat: 5.5 grams      (Carol W.)

"Make it taste good. Know what satisfies you—whether
soft or crunchy. A carload of lettuce won't satisfy you if
you want a cup of ice cream!" —Carol W.

♦ 3 ounces grilled mahimahi with lime juice
  ¾ cup cooked white rice with lemon pepper
  1 cup mixed vegetables (broccoli, cauliflower, carrots)
  1 small dinner roll
  1 cup mixed honeydew and cantaloupe cubes
      Calories: 477      Fat: 4 grams      (Pam W.)

◆ 3 ounces broiled or grilled pork tenderloin
½ cup mashed potatoes, made with skim milk
1 cup chopped broccoli, sprinkled with 1 teaspoon grated
  Parmesan cheese
Sliced Fruit Plate: ½ each small apple, banana and pear
8 ounces skim milk

    Calories: 492    Fat: 9 grams    (Linda W.)

> "I drink more milk now than I used to because I know
> my system needs it, but it is usually skim and never
> higher in fat than 1 percent." —Linda W.

◆ 4 baked chicken nuggets (3-ounce boneless chicken breast, cut
  into 4 pieces and dipped in ¼ cup buttermilk, then ¼ cup
  seasoned bread crumbs)
¾ cup cooked angel hair pasta with 1 tablespoon pesto and
  2 tablespoons sun-dried tomatoes
½ cup Italian green beans, steamed
1 slice watermelon (1-x-5-inch slice)

    Calories: 493    Fat: 11 grams    (Connye Z.)

> "Think! Is this really good?
> Is it worth the calories?" —Connye Z.

# 21 Snacks and Desserts from the Masters

## (100 calories or less)

◆ 2½ cups air-popped popcorn with 2 teaspoons grated Parmesan
  cheese

    Calories: 95    Fat: 2 grams    (Molly A.)

- 2 tablespoons semisweet chocolate chips

  Calories: 100    Fat: 6.5 grams                    (Thalia A.)

> "I include something that tastes really good each day." —Thalia A.

- 2 tablespoons candy corn

  Calories: 90    Fat: negligible                    (Patsy B.)

- 1 regular Fudgsicle (2.5-ounce) *or* 2 low-calorie Fudgsicles

  Calories: 91    Fat: negligible                    (Helen B.)

- 1 frozen yogurt bar (2.5-ounce)

  Calories: 100    Fat: 1 gram                    (Jane Brody)

- 1 cup frozen blueberries (still frozen!)

  Calories: 79    Fat: 1 gram                    (Cathy B.)

- ⅓ cup Cracklin' Oat Bran Cereal (dry)

  Calories: 76    Fat: 3 grams                    (Joy C.)

- 5 dried prunes (pitted)

  Calories: 100    Fat: negligible                    (Jennie C.)

- 25 fat-free baked potato chips

  Calories: 92    Fat: 0                    (Stephanie C.)

> "I caution people about fat-free snacks. They still add up calorically." —Stephanie C.

- 3 tablespoons raisins (try golden raisins for a change)
  Calories: 93          Fat: negligible          (Dorothy C.)

- 9 animal cookies
  Calories: 92          Fat: 3 grams          (Judy F.)

- 1 ounce red licorice
  Calories: 99          Fat: 0          (Shirley G.)

- 15 reduced-fat Wheat Thins
  Calories: 100          Fat: 3.5 grams          (Julie J.)

- 6 reduced-fat wheat crackers with 6 cucumber slices
  Calories: 100          Fat: 2.5 grams          (Cam L.)

- 18 tiny cinnamon cookies (such as SnackWell's Cinnamon Graham Stars)
  Calories: 99          Fat: 0          (Jean M.)

- Large Iced Coffee: 8 ounces skim milk, 1 cup strong coffee, 1 packet low-calorie sweetener (optional: add flavoring extracts, such as vanilla, rum, amaretto, almond or mint)
  Calories: 94          Fat: negligible          (Lynda M.)

  "Iced flavored coffee satisfies the sweet tooth." —Lynda M.

- 2 white Cheddar rice cakes
  Calories: 80          Fat: 0          (Joanna M.)

"When I have a craving, I try to substitute
something low-fat but similar in texture or taste.
For example, if I want potato chips,
I might eat rice cakes." —Joanna M.

◆ 1-ounce slice warm sourdough bread, spread with honey-Dijon
mustard
Calories: 94          Fat: 2 grams          (Renee R.)

◆ 2 plain rice cakes topped with ¼ cup unsweetened applesauce and
sprinkled with cinnamon
Calories: 96          Fat: negligible          (Jim V.)

◆ 1 large, juicy navel orange (7-ounce)
Calories: 92          Fat: negligible          (Linda W.)

◆ ¾ cup dry Trix cereal
Calories: 81          Fat: negligible          (Arlene Z.)

# 21 Snacks and Desserts from the Masters

### (200 calories or less)

◆ 1½-ounce slice low-fat pound cake, topped with ⅓ cup fresh
sliced strawberries and ¼ cup fat-free strawberry frozen yogurt
Calories: 190          Fat: 2.5 grams          (Thalia A.)

◆ 6-ounce glass dry white wine
½-ounce reduced-fat Cheddar cheese
2 reduced-fat wheat crackers
>   Calories: 192       Fat: 3.5 grams                    (Celia G.)


◆ Baked sweet potato (5-ounce), sliced and microwaved with ⅓ cup
miniature marshmallows on top
>   Calories: 196       Fat: negligible                    (Dorothy C.)


◆ 1 cup sugar-free hot cocoa, made from a mix
4 zwieback toasts
>   Calories: 183       Fat: 3.5 grams                    (Maxine D.)

> "Don't give up if you gain one week;
> the next week, you will lose." —Maxine D.


◆ Cinnamon Toast: 2 slices reduced-calorie wheat toast, 2 teaspoons
margarine, 2 teaspoons cinnamon sugar
>   Calories: 189       Fat: 9 grams                    (Judy F.)


◆ 2-ounce piece angel food cake with ½ cup fresh sliced strawberries
and 2 tablespoons reduced-fat dessert topping
>   Calories: 191       Fat: 2 grams                    (Ann F.)

> "Find low-fat substitutes: angel food cake
> for chocolate cake, gingersnaps for Oreos,
> low-fat crackers." —Ann F.


◆ 1¼ cups nonfat sugar-free frozen yogurt
>   Calories: 188       Fat: 0                    (Stan J.)

♦ 20 reduced-fat taco chips with ⅓ cup salsa
  Calories: 191     Fat: 2 grams              (Gaylord J.)


♦ 2-ounce soft pretzel (unsalted) with 2 teaspoons mustard
  Calories: 198     Fat: 2 grams              (Mary Ann K.)


♦ 1 cup fresh strawberries
  9 pretzel twists
  Calories: 197     Fat: 2.5 grams            (Cam L.)


♦ 1¼ cups nonfat, sugar-free chocolate pudding *or* ¾ cup nonfat
  pudding, sweetened with sugar
  Calories: 196     Fat: negligible           (Don Mauer)


♦ 1 cup sugar-free strawberry gelatin
  3 fat-free fig bars
  Calories: 166     Fat: 0                    (Jacque M.)


♦ Curried Popcorn: 4 cups air-popped popcorn tossed with
  ½ tablespoon olive oil and seasoned with curry powder and salt
  Calories: 185     Fat: 8 grams              (Gail O.)


♦ 6 reduced-fat cinnamon crisp graham cracker squares with
  2 tablespoons nonfat cream cheese
  Calories: 195     Fat: 2.5 grams            (Emil R.)


♦ 1 ounce (3 tablespoons) shelled peanuts
  Calories: 160     Fat: 13.5 grams           (Lorene N.)

- ⅔ cup chocolate chip cookie dough "lite" ice cream in a plain cone

  Calories: 200     Fat: 5 grams        (Marlene R.)

- 6 low-fat wheat crackers spread with ¼ ripe avocado

  Calories: 178     Fat: 10 grams       (Renee R.)

- Baked Apple: Microwave 1 medium apple stuffed with 2 tablespoons raisins and sprinkled with cinnamon; Serve with 3 tablespoons fat-free vanilla yogurt

  Calories: 188     Fat: negligible      (Edith S.)

  > "I try to find satisfying substitutes.
  > I used to love apple pie. Now, the above
  > combination works for me." —Edith S.

- 1¾ cups fat-free caramel popcorn

  Calories: 193     Fat: 0           (Beth W.)

- 8 ounces nonfat plain yogurt with ⅔ cup frozen blueberries, 2 packets low-calorie sweetener (or to taste), nutmeg and cinnamon (Bob says, "This tastes like blueberry-yogurt ice cream.")

  Calories: 195     Fat: 1.5 grams       (Bob W.)

- 2¾-ounce slice reduced-fat chocolate cake (Connye likes Weight Watchers Double Fudge Cake.)

  Calories: 190     Fat: 4.5 grams       (Connye Z.)

# Free Foods

**Beverages:** water, sugar-free soft drinks, carbonated water, black coffee or tea

**Flavoring agents:** low-calorie sugar substitutes (aspartame, saccharin), low-calorie butter-flavoring products, lemon or lime juice, flavoring extracts (vanilla, almond, etc.), herbs and spices, horseradish, marinades (not as a sauce, just to marinate foods), soy or Worcestershire sauce (high in sodium), mustard, vinegar, garlic

**Miscellaneous:** nonstick cooking spray, sugar-free gum (up to 5 sticks per day), unsweetened pickles (high in sodium)

AFTER THE DIET IS DONE:

# How the Masters Make the Transition to a New Way of Eating

ONCE YOU HAVE FINALLY ARRIVED AT A COMFORTABLE WEIGHT, the next step to a new food life is making the transition out of the weight-loss plan and into maintenance. During this pivotal time, you go from eating less food to eating more—but just the right amount to maintain your new weight.

The transition to maintenance is the most difficult time for dieters. Kay D. speaks for many masters: "If I was ever going to fail, it was going to be now. It was almost like being kicked out of a nest—you've got your wings, now go on out there and fly."

Many masters admit that making the transition was largely a trial-and-error process. As Stephanie C. (27 pounds, 18 years) explains, "I had to find what worked and what didn't. Sometimes I would look at a full plate of food, and after eating it, I would think, 'My God, all that large portion of food is now inside of ME.' That would help me cut down on portions."

How much more you can eat during maintenance depends on how restrictive your weight-loss plan was, on your own individual calorie needs and on how much you exercise. When I asked the masters how many daily calories they figure they consume now at maintenance, the range was widespread: from 1,000 to more than 2,100. Although there is no way to be certain in advance what foods you can eat once you reach your goal, the masters used the following techniques to make the transition out of the diet stage and into the keep-it-off-forever state of maintenance.

**Eat more of what you're already eating.** This option works well if you lose weight with a nondieting approach or a sensible low-calorie food plan. Until your weight levels off, you experiment by slowly increasing amounts of foods you're already eating. Paul A. (46 pounds, 5 years) says, "It was a difficult transition. I had to tell myself that I must eat the same foods—only a bit more. I followed the Weight Watchers plan, adding foods until my weight stabilized."

Janice G. (30 pounds, 13 years) recalls, "I added slowly, starting with two slices of toast in place of one at breakfast, keeping in mind that 100 calories too many per day equals a 10-pound gain in a year."

For some masters, the transition to maintenance went so smoothly that they felt as though they were continuing to do exactly what they had done while losing. *In fact, 25 percent of the masters say that their food habits are no different at maintenance than they were when they were losing weight.*

**Let the scale guide you.** Regardless of how they lost the weight, many masters weighed themselves regularly while easing into maintenance. Beth W. says that after she lost her 73 pounds, "I watched the scale and went by how my clothes fit. If I felt myself creeping back up, I started to watch what I ate and exercised more. I never let myself gain more than 5 pounds."

The masters use the scale to see whether their new food lives are working and to determine whether they need to make some adjustments. Most of them don't seem to be slaves to it but matter-of-factly use the information to guide daily food choices. Most establish a weight "buffer zone"—a maximum upper limit, usually not more than 5 to 10 pounds above what they feel is their optimal weight. If they gain more than that, they take action.

**Get support.** Many masters who lost their weight with the help of a program stressed the importance of continuing to get support at the maintenance stage. *Research suggests that sticking with a program until you meet your goal and well into maintenance can be critical for long-term success.* Like other masters, Kay D. and Stan J., profiled in Chapters One and Two respectively, were involved in the maintenance part of their program far longer than in the actual weight-loss phase. And they, along with a number of long-term masters, still go back periodically for support. It appears that continuing to be involved in a maintenance program is particularly important for people who have lost weight as part of a strict diet program.

**Add a few treats.** Debbie T. says, "I cut out sweets when I was in the process of losing my weight. Once I reached my goal, I added a sweet once in a while as a special treat." (See Chapter Four, "If You Want It, Have It.") Joy C. says that as she eased into maintenance, she allowed herself a few treats on weekends and was more careful on the other five days.

**Trash your large-sized clothes.** A number of masters say that it helps to get rid of your old, big clothes. JoAnna L. explains, "I got rid of all my clothing that became too large. Having bigger sizes to fall back on was always a crutch in the past. It really was a self-fulfilling prophecy."

**Keep track of what you eat.** Some masters emphasized the importance of formally keeping tabs on what they ate as they made the transition to maintenance. Jennifer B. notes, "Food diaries helped so I could find out what calorie range I could allow myself without gaining." In fact, research studies suggest that people who keep track of what they eat lose more weight and are more likely to keep it off than are those who don't.

*The majority of masters—3 out of every 4—still record what they eat, at least occasionally.* They do so in several ways: by keeping food diaries, writing down everything they eat; by counting calories and/or fat grams; by monitoring food groups. Quite a few just keep track mentally, and a number find it particularly helpful to go back to writing foods down when they're having trouble. Of those who keep track on occasion, JoAnna L. writes down what she eats only one day a week. "Six of the seven days, I just go on 'cruise control,' but the one day a week that I'm accountable to myself keeps the other six from going out of control."

**Balance food and exercise.** The subject of exercise came up repeatedly when I asked the masters how they eased into a maintenance way of life. *Exercise allows you to eat more and provides damage control*—a number of masters use exercise to offset dietary indiscretions. Patsy K. advises, "When you know you have consumed too many calories, make it a point to do some extra activity to burn off some of the extra calories." Exercise also makes people feel good and can help temper the desire to turn to food for comfort.

Many people are relieved to find that most masters are not exercise fanatics—only 35 of the 208 exercise every day. The majority do, however, exercise more than most people: 3 out of 4 masters exercise at least three times a week; 70 of the masters exercise three to four times a week, while 54 of them work out five or six times weekly. For most masters, the exercise of choice is walking—129 of them are walkers. Other popular forms of exercise with the masters are cycling (stationary or mobile), aerobics, lifting light weights and jogging. Quite a few use a ski machine or stair climber, swim, rollerblade or do calisthenics. Finally, the masters tend to vary their exercise: 6 out of 10 engage in at least two different forms, such as walking and cycling.

# Make a Lifelong Commitment

**M**AKING THE TRANSITION from losing weight to maintenance can be unnerving, but the masters have weathered it. Kay D., who says that reaching her goal was one of the scariest days of her life, explains how she made it through the transition: "I learned new habits the whole time I was dieting. During maintenance, I continued to make healthy choices using lessons learned while losing."

Kay D. is describing how she, like so many other masters, began to see that she couldn't go back to her old ways. In fact, when I asked the masters, "How do you think your eating habits are different from those of people who lose weight and gain weight back?" their most common responses had to do with lifestyle change and realizing that they cannot return to their old habits.

Here's how Kay sums it up, "I made a *lifetime* commitment to changing to good habits and eating the proper foods. After losing, I did not slip back to my old ways of viewing food." Shirley G. elaborates, "Most people think they can go back to their former eating habits, which made them fat in the first place. You can't do this. You can allow a few more treats and eat a few larger meals on special occasions, but you must still watch it at other times." (Shirley's "watching it" for the past 20 years has enabled her to keep off 85 pounds.)

In essence, I found a matter-of-fact acceptance among the masters of the need for a permanent new way of living, thinking and eating, as illustrated by 18-year master Karen S., who states, "Acceptance of a lifestyle change is essential. I didn't want to spend the rest of my life hating myself. I made up my mind that in order to stay thinner, I'd always have to exercise and eat relatively carefully. It is worth it to me." Hazel U. adds, "I do not consider myself 'dieting' or 'on a diet.' I feel that I must keep eating this way for the rest of my life to stay thin and healthy. My eating habits have changed for life."

# PART III

# EATING THIN *for* LIFE Recipes

*122 Favorites
from the Masters*

CHAPTER SEVEN

# Learn to Cook a New Way

**E**N ROUTE TO THEIR NEW FOOD LIVES, most of the masters learned to cook a new way, experimenting and coming up with a low-fat style of cooking that makes eating pleasurable. As Diane J. explained over and over again, "*Everything* is about taste. We can be satisfied with fewer fat grams if the food tastes good." *The masters have discovered how to create low-fat fare that is still full of flavor.*

## Diane J.'s Story

**L**IKE A NUMBER OF HER FELLOW MASTERS, Diane is an avid low-fat cooking hobbyist and delights in coming up with new recipes almost every day. And it pays off—Diane is an attractive, stately 5'9" 58-year-old who looks as though she weighs even less than her 169 pounds—43 pounds shy of her all-time high.

Diane has always been a good cook, but for a long time, her cooking was bad news for her weight problem. "We ate many gravies and cheeses; anything I could put cheese on, I did—I'd add two cups to macaroni and cheese or to au gratin potatoes. We also loved blue cheese dressing, but not the bottled kind. I asked a chef in a local restaurant for his recipe, and it made more than four gallons! Several friends and I would get together, make the recipe and split it up. My husband and I would put blue cheese dressing on everything; we dipped French fries in it, put it on baked potatoes, salads. All I used was butter—in cookies, on vegetables, on toast. I also did a lot of deep-fat frying."

After her lifestyle landed her at the doctor's office weighing more than 200 pounds and complaining of chest pains, Diane made a commitment to cook differently. She began to "take baby steps," changing one small habit at a time. She explains, "The first thing we did was to go from 2 percent to 1 percent milk. Oh, the complaining! But we handled it. Once we got used to that, I started mixing skim and 1 percent milk. Now, we drink only skim."

The next step Diane took was to cut back on the red meat she served. "At first, it was hard to cut back—my husband felt deprived," she says. "If we could get by with two dinners a week without meat, it was a big accomplishment. Now, we have red meat twice a week, at the most. If we feel like cooking steak, we have swordfish—it tastes like beef to us, but it's better." The next thing to go was processed meat. "We looked at all the bologna and knockwurst we were eating and that went too. Now, when we want something like this, we use Canadian bacon instead."

All the while that Diane was imposing her "baby steps" on her protesting husband and adapting her favorite recipes, she was learning how to be an excellent low-fat cook. "I couldn't serve him cardboard-flavored foods and expect him to say, 'This is really good.'

"I learned early on that when you take out the fat, you have to put something back in. For flavor, I started playing around with spices, garlic, onion, herbs and nonfat seasonings. I discovered that I could get a butter taste with Molly McButter. With Molly McCheese, I could get a cheese taste." She continues to experiment with low-fat products, like reduced-fat cheeses and nonfat cooking sprays.

Diane's philosophy is: "You take out, you put back in." She explains, "When I make muffins, I ask myself, 'How can I do away with butter or oil and still keep them moist?' I learned that you can cut the oil and add applesauce or crushed pineapple. To make up for flavor loss, I might add nutmeg and cinnamon. If a recipe calls for milk or cream, I use skim milk and add butter flavoring. In place of eggs, I use Egg Beaters." Although she works hard to shave fat and calories from recipes, she notes, "You don't have to cut everything out." For instance, she occasionally uses butter, but "sparingly." And she sometimes adds a little bacon fat or bacon to a recipe, "because it imparts such good flavor." (For more ideas, see "Tricks of the Low-Fat Cooking Trade," page 144.)

# TRICKS OF THE LOW-FAT COOKING TRADE

### Keep baked goods tender and moist

♦ When cutting fat, substitute an equal amount of mashed or pureed fruit—baby food works fine. Applesauce can be substituted for all or some of the oil in many recipes. (Apples contain pectin, which prevents moisture loss during baking.) Pureed prunes are also good fat substitutes, particularly in chocolate-flavored baked goods. Use baby-food prunes, or puree pitted prunes with some hot water in a blender.

♦ Buttermilk is a good moistening agent, because it has more body than other liquids.

♦ Use undiluted juice concentrates for extra moistening and flavor.

♦ To bring out sweetness, increase the vanilla extract.

### Add "savor flavor" to your favorite dishes

♦ Instead of heavy sauces, add more herbs and spices.

♦ Use more salsa and hot sauces.

♦ Be heavy-handed with members of the onion family, including regular onions, red onions, green onions and leeks.

♦ Discover flavored vinegars for salad dressings. Instead of 3 parts oil to 1 part vinegar, switch to 3 parts vinegar, 1 part oil.

◆ Add grated, pureed or finely chopped vegetables to sauces and to recipes with higher-fat ingredients: Put grated carrots in meat loaf, and add finely chopped peppers, onions and celery to meatless spaghetti sauce.

◆ Add nonfat relishes to egg or tuna salads.

### Reduce fat, boost flavor

◆ Use small amounts of flavored oils, such as olive, sesame and walnut, because their unique taste goes a long way.

◆ Use powdered butter substitutes or nonfat butter sprays instead of butter on steamed vegetables and mashed potatoes.

◆ For a flavorful high-fat item, such as chopped nuts or bacon, cut the amount by one-half to three-fourths.

◆ Try nonfat yogurt in place of some of the oil or mayonnaise.

◆ Use skim milk in recipes calling for whole milk. Substitute evaporated skim milk for cream.

◆ Use reduced-fat and nonfat cheeses in place of regular. A single ounce of many cheeses has more than 8 grams of fat. Experiment, since some low-fat kinds are better than others. Reduced-fat types taste and melt better than nonfat. Be aware that the fat can add up, so go easy.

◆ Use small amounts of intensely flavored cheeses, such as Parmesan or blue cheese.

◆ Use nonfat ricotta, cottage cheese or sour cream in place of regular.

◆ Puree nonfat or low-fat cottage cheese in a blender or a food processor until smooth, then use it in place of all or part of the cream cheese and sour cream.

◆ When a recipe calls for cream soup, substitute one can of low-fat or fat-free chicken noodle soup pureed in a blender.

◆ When using fat-free cream cheese in cooking, mix in 1 tablespoon of cornstarch per 8-ounce block to keep the cream cheese from separating in the cooking process.

### Always choose the best

◆ Buy the best flavored vinegars and the finest Dijon mustard.

◆ Use pure vanilla extract rather than imitation.

◆ Crush or grate garlic by hand instead of using powder.

◆ Use fresh herbs in place of dried, increasing the amount by three times.

◆ Grind pepper in a pepper mill rather than using commercial ground pepper.

◆ Grate your own nutmeg with a grater.

◆ Use fresh-squeezed lemon and lime juice instead of bottled.

### Remember to make it look nice— eye appeal adds no fat.

Within 1½ years, Diane had reached her goal of 170 pounds. She had also won her husband over to her low-fat recipes, and he lost 79 pounds. Now, when Diane feels like she's not in control of her eating, she returns to her favorite sources of inspiration. "I get into the bathtub with a bunch of cookbooks and look at recipes. I think, 'What can I do to power this down, fatwise?'"

# Getting Started in the Kitchen

IF, LIKE DIANE J., you've prepared food a certain way for many years, it can seem a daunting task to learn how to cook all over again. But you don't have to do it all at once. The easiest place to start is with your favorite recipes, paring down the amount of fat they call for by one-half, then cutting back even more if that works.

JoAnna L. advises, "You have to zero in on the types of foods you have always loved. Then, go out and find good low-fat and low-sugar alternatives to those foods. If you don't eat the types of foods you feel comfortable with, then your new eating habits will be short-lived. If you like Mexican, then fix healthy Mexican. If you like dessert, as I do, then make sure you have some type of healthy dessert every day." JoAnna has used her philosophy to bring about a 130-pound weight loss and to become a successful author and publisher of healthful recipes. Bob W. (246 pounds, 23 years) urges: "Go to cooking classes. Buy *Cooking Light* and *Eating Well* magazines."

You certainly don't have to spend your life becoming a low-fat gourmet. Brad H. suggests, "Learn five new low-fat recipes, and cook them instead of your favorites."

On the road to becoming an accomplished low-fat cook, Diane J. admits that she has had a few disasters, which she considers all part of the learning process. "When low-fat baked goods flop, you have to throw them away. But I can always salvage foods like soup by adding things to them." Don Mauer, another accomplished low-fat cook, puts his mistakes into perspective too: "The worst thing that can happen is that you'll have to throw away what you made. But you'll also be one step closer to success."

# About the Recipes

I F YOU ARE ON A LOW-SODIUM OR OTHER SPECIAL DIET, you should check with your physician and a dietitian before using the following recipes, since their emphasis is on lowering fat and calories, not sodium. Many of the recipes, however, can be easily adapted by omitting added salt, using fresh rather than canned products and using reduced- or low-sodium versions of products like spaghetti sauce and broth.

◆ Nonstick cooking spray is used in many of the following recipes and is not mentioned in the ingredient list, nor is it included in the nutrition analyses.

◆ Egg substitutes should be fat-free. (Check labels.)

◆ Reduced-fat cheeses used in these recipes should have no more than 5 grams of fat per ounce. (For purposes of analysis, reduced-fat cheeses with 5 grams of fat per ounce were used.)

◆ Diet margarine used is 50 percent lower in fat than regular margarine, unless otherwise indicated.

◆ Extra-lean hamburger refers to packages stating "90 percent lean."

◆ Weights of bell peppers used are as follows: small (3 ounces), medium (6 ounces), large (9 ounces).

◆ Weights of onions used are as follows: small (2-3 ounces), medium (3-4 ounces), large (5-6 ounces).

◆ Ground turkey is from boneless, skinless turkey breast. (Ask the supermarket butcher to grind it, or grind it yourself.)

◆ Whenever beef or chicken broth is used, be sure to skim any fat off the top.

◆ Parmesan cheese is shredded rather than grated. Shredded is coarser than grated and can be purchased at the grocery store in the cheese section.

◆ Sodium values for recipes calling for cooked pasta products do not include salt added to the cooking water, because the amount of sodium depends on how heavy-handed you are with the salt shaker.

# About the Nutritional Analyses

IN THE FOLLOWING RECIPES, nutrition information is provided for a single serving.

● Optional ingredients are not included in the analyses.

● If a choice of ingredients is offered, such as "margarine or butter," the first item was used for the analysis.

● If a range of servings is listed, the analysis applies to the smaller serving size; that is, for a serving of 6 to 8, the analysis would be for 8 servings.

● When a range is given for an ingredient, the average was analyzed.

# Breads and Breakfast Fare

# Pineapple Right-Side-Up Coffee Cake

*Gaylord J.*

SERVES 10

IT'S HARD TO BELIEVE that anything this easy and this low in fat can taste so good! It's moist and rich-tasting—a real winner as a breakfast bread or for dessert. (If you want, at the same time that you add the pineapple, you can also add ¼ cup raisins, chopped dates or chopped apricots.)

|       |                                                              |
|-------|--------------------------------------------------------------|
| 2½    | cups all-purpose flour                                       |
| 1½    | cups granulated sugar                                        |
| ¼     | cup light or dark brown sugar                                |
| 1     | teaspoon baking soda                                         |
| ½     | teaspoon baking powder                                       |
| ½     | teaspoon salt                                                |
| ⅓     | cup pecan or walnut halves (about 1.3 ounces), chopped       |
| 1     | can (20 ounces) crushed pineapple in its own juice           |

1. Preheat oven to 375 degrees F, with a rack in center. Coat bottom and sides of a 9-to-10-inch springform pan with nonstick cooking spray. Set aside.

2. In a large bowl, stir together all dry ingredients, including nuts, until well mixed.

3. Add pineapple and juice. Stir gently with a wooden spoon just until moistened; do not overmix. Pour into prepared pan.

4. Bake for 50 to 55 minutes, or until a toothpick inserted in center comes out clean. Cool for 10 minutes on a wire rack. Run a knife around edges of pan to loosen. Release sides and continue cooling. Serve warm, at room temperature or chilled.

PER SERVING: CALORIES: 304; FAT: 3 G; CHOLESTEROL: 0 MG; SODIUM: 260 MG; PROTEIN: 4 G; CARBOHYDRATE: 67 G

# Hawaiian Yeast Bread

*Cindy P.*

MAKES 3 LOAVES, 12 THICK SLICES PER LOAF

PINEAPPLE JUICE AND GINGER work together to give each slice of this bread a sweet—but not too sweet—spicy flavor, making it easy to forgo butter. And because of its rich, dense texture—conferred by instant mashed potato flakes, which are kneaded in with the flour—you feel satisfied with one or two slices. This bread is perfect for breakfast or brunch or at suppertime with a fruit salad and cottage cheese. (The recipe makes 3 loaves, so it's well worth the effort.)

|   |   |
|---|---|
| 6 | cups all-purpose flour, plus 1-2 cups more for kneading |
| ⅔ | cup granulated sugar |
| ¾ | cup instant mashed potato flakes |
| 2 | envelopes active dry yeast |
| 1 | teaspoon salt |
| ½ | teaspoon ground ginger |
| 1 | cup unsweetened pineapple juice |
| 3 | large egg whites |
| 2 | teaspoons vanilla extract |
| 1 | cup skim milk |
| ½ | cup water |
| 4 | tablespoons (½ stick) margarine |

1. Spray 3 loaf pans (9 x 5 x 3 inches or 8½ x 4½ x 2½ inches) with nonstick cooking spray. In a large mixing bowl, stir together 3 cups flour, sugar, potato flakes, yeast, salt and ginger. Set aside.

2. In a small bowl, with a wire whisk, blend together juice, egg whites and vanilla. Set aside.

3. In a small saucepan over medium heat, combine milk, water and margarine. Heat to 105 to 115 degrees F, or until very warm (but not hot) and margarine melts, stirring occasionally.

4. Add milk mixture to dry ingredients. Add juice mixture and beat with a heavy-duty electric mixer or a wooden spoon until smooth. Add 3 more cups of flour, 1 cup at a time, until dough pulls away from sides of bowl and is easy to handle.

5. Turn out onto a lightly floured surface. Knead until smooth and elastic, about 10 minutes, adding more flour as needed. Place dough in a large bowl sprayed with nonstick cooking spray. Cover with plastic wrap that has been sprayed with nonstick cooking spray. Let rise at room temperature or in a warm place until doubled in size, or until an indentation remains when bread is pressed slightly with a fingertip, approximately 2 hours.

6. Punch down dough; divide into thirds. Shape into loaves and place in prepared loaf pans. Cover with plastic wrap that has been sprayed with nonstick cooking spray and let rise until doubled in size.

7. When ready to bake, preheat oven to 350 degrees F, with a rack in center. Bake until loaves are golden brown and sound hollow when tapped, 25 to 30 minutes. Remove loaves from pans and let cool on a wire rack. Serve warm or at room temperature. (To freeze, cool completely and wrap tightly.)

PER SLICE: CALORIES: 133; FAT: 1.5 G; CHOLESTEROL: 0 MG; SODIUM: 84 MG; PROTEIN: 3 G; CARBOHYDRATE: 26 G

# Mediterranean Herb Bread

*Cathy B.*

MAKES 2 LOAVES, ABOUT 20 SLICES PER LOAF

THIS YEAST BREAD is stuffed with pesto (a blend of olive oil, basil and garlic), giving it a pinwheel effect when it is sliced. The moist, flavorful herb filling eliminates the need for butter and makes the bread the perfect accompaniment for any type of pasta. Cathy always likes to add a little gluten flour, because she feels it makes the bread dough more elastic and because the finished bread is less likely to be crumbly. (Gluten, or starch-free wheat flour, can be purchased in regular supermarkets or natural-food stores.) You can omit the gluten flour and increase the amount of all-purpose flour to 6½ cups.

DOUGH
1   tablespoon active dry yeast
2   tablespoons granulated sugar
2   cups warm water (105-115 degrees F)
1½  teaspoons salt
¼   cup gluten flour
6   cups all-purpose flour

HERB FILLING
1¾  cups fresh basil leaves
⅓   cup fresh parsley leaves
⅓   cup shredded Parmesan cheese
⅓   cup olive oil
3   large garlic cloves
¾   teaspoon salt

1. **To make dough:** In a large bowl, combine yeast, sugar and water. Let stand for 5 to 10 minutes, or until yeast starts to foam.

2. With a wooden spoon or a heavy-duty electric mixer, stir in salt, then flours, 1 cup at a time, until a smooth dough forms and pulls away from sides of bowl.

3. Turn dough out onto a lightly floured board and knead for about 10 minutes, or until smooth and elastic. (If your electric mixer has a dough hook, knead for 5 minutes on medium speed.)

4. Place dough in a clean bowl generously sprayed with nonstick cooking spray. Turn to coat lightly all over. Cover and let rise in a warm, draft-free place until dough has doubled in size, 1 to 2 hours.

5. **To make herb filling**: In a food processor fitted with the metal blade or in a blender, process all ingredients until smooth. Set aside.

6. Turn out dough onto a lightly floured surface and divide in half. Knead each half for about 2 minutes, or until smooth. Roll each half into a rectangle approximately 10 x 12 inches. Spread half of herb filling over each rectangle, leaving a 1-inch margin all around. Starting at the shorter end, roll dough up tightly, jellyroll-style. Pinch seams and ends well to seal them. Pat each roll into a loaf shape. Transfer loaves, seam side down, to a cookie sheet coated with nonstick cooking spray. Cover with a kitchen towel. Allow loaves to rise for ½ to 1 hour, or until one-fourth to one-third larger. Preheat oven to 375 degrees F.

7. Slash top of each loaf with a razor-sharp knife or kitchen shears, making 4 or 5 diagonal cuts ½ inch deep. Bake for 30 minutes, or until loaves are golden brown and sound hollow when tapped. Cool on a wire rack for about 15 minutes before serving.

PER SLICE: CALORIES: 94; FAT: 2 G; CHOLESTEROL: 0 MG; SODIUM: 132 MG; PROTEIN: 3 G; CARBOHYDRATE: 16 G

# Tom's Onion Bagels

### *Tom F.*

##### MAKES 16 BAGELS

THESE MAKE GREAT SNACK FOOD when eaten plain and warm, or use them to make a sandwich. (Try smoked turkey breast, Dijon-style mustard and lettuce.) You can intensify the flavor by sprinkling a little onion powder on top of each bagel before baking.

|       |                                          |
|-------|------------------------------------------|
| 1     | envelope active dry yeast                |
| 1     | tablespoon granulated sugar              |
| 1½    | teaspoons salt                           |
| 2     | cups warm water (105-115 degrees F)      |
| 6-6½  | cups all-purpose flour                   |
| 1     | large onion, finely chopped (about ¾ cup)|

1. Spray 2 cookie sheets with nonstick cooking spray. Set aside.

2. In a large bowl, mix yeast, sugar, salt and water. Let stand for 5 to 10 minutes, or until yeast starts to foam. Add 3 cups flour, 1 cup at a time, mixing well with a wooden spoon after each addition. Mix in onion. Add 2 more cups flour, 1 cup at a time, mixing well after each addition. (Dough will pull away from sides of bowl and feel a little sticky.) Remove dough and set aside. Place dough in a clean bowl generously sprayed with nonstick cooking spray and cover with plastic wrap coated with nonstick cooking spray. Let rise in a warm, draft-free place until doubled in size, about 2 hours.

3. After dough has doubled, punch it down. Turn out onto a lightly floured surface and knead for about 15 minutes, or until dough is smooth and has a satiny appearance. (If it is too sticky to handle, add 1 tablespoon flour at a time until it is easy to work.)

4. Form dough into 16 balls about the size of golf balls, and push your floured thumb through the center of each to create a ring about 3½ inches across. Evenly space rings on cookie sheets. Cover with kitchen towels and refrigerate for 20 minutes. Remove from refrigerator and let rise for 20 minutes in a warm, draft-free place until slightly puffed.

5. Preheat oven to 425 degrees F. Bring 3 to 4 quarts water to a boil in a wide 4-to-6-quart pan. Slide bagels in, 4 at a time. Boil for 4 minutes, turning 3 to 4 times. Remove with a slotted spoon and drain on a towel. Arrange on cookie sheets, making sure bagels do not touch.

6. Bake bagels for 25 to 30 minutes, or until golden brown. Transfer to a wire rack and cool slightly. Serve warm.

PER BAGEL: CALORIES: 185; FAT: 0.5 G; CHOLESTEROL: 0 MG; SODIUM: 202 MG; PROTEIN: 5 G; CARBOHYDRATE: 39 G

# Carrot Muffins with Orange Glaze

*Diane J.*

MAKES 12 MUFFINS

GREAT FOR BREAKFAST, these muffins can also be served as a dessert cupcake. If you want to skip the glaze, Diane suggests spraying the cooked muffins with a light coating of butter-flavored nonstick spray and sprinkling them with a mixture of cinnamon and sugar.

MUFFINS

2 tablespoons butter or margarine, softened
¾ cup granulated sugar
1 teaspoon vanilla extract
1 large egg
2 large egg whites
2 cups shredded carrots (about 4 medium)
1 teaspoon grated orange rind
¼ cup skim milk
1 cup all-purpose flour
½ cup uncooked quick-cooking oatmeal
1¼ teaspoons baking powder
1 teaspoon ground cinnamon
¾ teaspoon baking soda
½ teaspoon ground nutmeg
¼ teaspoon salt

GLAZE

¾ cup powdered sugar
1 tablespoon orange juice
¼ teaspoon grated orange rind

1. **To make muffins:** Preheat oven to 350 degrees F. Spray a 12-cup muffin pan with nonstick cooking spray or use paper cupcake liners. Set aside.

2. In a medium mixing bowl, with an electric mixer on medium-low speed, cream butter or margarine and sugar until smooth, then mix in vanilla. Add egg and egg whites, one at a time, beating well after each addition. Stir in carrots, orange rind and milk. Set aside.

3. In a large bowl, stir together dry ingredients.

4. Pour liquid ingredients over dry ingredients. Stir by hand just until blended; do not overmix.

5. Spoon batter into prepared muffin pan, filling each cup about three-fourths full. Bake until muffins are lightly browned and a toothpick inserted in center comes out clean, about 20 to 25 minutes. Cool slightly in pans. Turn out and cool on a wire rack.

6. **To make glaze:** Just before serving, mix powdered sugar, orange juice and rind by hand in a small bowl. Spoon a small amount on top of each muffin. If you want a thinner glaze, add more orange juice, one drop at a time; if you want a thicker glaze, add more powdered sugar, 1 tablespoon at a time.

PER MUFFIN: CALORIES: 167; FAT: 2.5 G; CHOLESTEROL: 23 MG; SODIUM: 251 MG; PROTEIN: 3 G; CARBOHYDRATE: 33 G

# Cinnamon-Apple Muffins

*Gaylord J.*

MAKES ABOUT 28 MUFFINS

LMOST LIKE CAKE, these muffins are moist and full of apple flavor. They're great for breakfast or to head off an evening sweettooth attack. The recipe makes a large quantity, so you can freeze part of the batch.

2    cups all-purpose flour
1    cup uncooked quick-cooking oatmeal
2    rounded tablespoons ground cinnamon
3    teaspoons baking powder
1    teaspoon baking soda
½    teaspoon salt
2    cups granulated sugar
1    cup skim milk
⅓    cup (5⅓ tablespoons) butter or margarine,
     softened
1    large egg
2    large apples, such as Granny Smith
     (about 20 ounces total weight),
     chopped into ¼-inch pieces

1. Preheat oven to 350 degrees F. Spray muffin pans with nonstick cooking spray or use paper cupcake liners. Set aside. (Note that this recipe makes about 28 muffins. If you don't have enough muffin pans to make this many at once, bake in separate batches.)

2. In a large bowl, stir together flour, oatmeal, cinnamon, baking powder, baking soda and salt. Set aside.

3. In another large bowl, whisk together sugar, milk, butter or margarine and egg until thoroughly blended. Whisk in apples.

4. Pour liquid ingredients over dry ingredients. With a wooden spoon or a rubber spatula, stir just until blended. Be careful not to overmix.

5. Spoon batter into prepared muffin pans, filling each cup about three-fourths full. Bake for 20 to 25 minutes, or until a toothpick inserted in center comes out clean. Cool slightly in pans. Turn out and cool on wire racks before serving.

PER MUFFIN: CALORIES: 134; FAT: 2.5 G; CHOLESTEROL: 14 MG; SODIUM: 194 MG; PROTEIN: 2 G; CARBOHYDRATE: 26 G

# Raspberry-Banana Bran Muffins

*Barbara M.*

MAKES 36 MUFFINS

BANANAS AND RASPBERRIES work together to make these muffins moist and low in fat. This recipe yields a large quantity, some of which can be frozen.

| | |
|---|---|
| 2 | tablespoons apple cider vinegar |
| 2 | cups skim milk |
| 1½ | cups all-purpose flour |
| 1½ | cups whole wheat flour |
| ¾ | cup granulated sugar |
| ⅓ | cup light or dark brown sugar |
| 2½ | teaspoons baking soda |
| 3 | cups Bran Buds cereal |
| 1 | cup boiling water |
| 1 | cup mashed very ripe banana (about 2 medium or 11-12 ounces before peeling) |
| ⅓ | cup vegetable oil |
| 2 | teaspoons vanilla extract |
| ½ | cup (4-ounce carton) egg substitute, thawed, or 4 large egg whites |
| 2 | cups frozen unsweetened raspberries, thawed and well drained |

1. Preheat oven to 350 degrees F. Spray muffin pans with nonstick cooking spray or use paper cupcake liners. Set aside. (Note that this recipe makes 36 muffins. If you don't have enough muffin pans to make this many at once, bake in separate batches.)

2. In a medium bowl, stir together vinegar and milk. (Milk will sour and curdle.) Set aside for 5 minutes, or until ready to use.

3. In another medium bowl, stir together flours, sugars and baking soda. Set aside.

4. Put Bran Buds in a large bowl. Pour boiling water over and stir gently just until water is absorbed. Set aside.

5. Add banana, oil, vanilla and egg substitute or whites to sour milk, then stir into Bran Buds.

6. Gently stir liquid ingredients into dry ingredients; do not over-mix. Fold in raspberries.

7. Spoon batter into prepared muffin pans, filling each cup about three-fourths full. Bake for 15 to 20 minutes, or until tops are golden and bounce back when touched lightly. Remove from pans immediately and allow to cool on wire racks.

PER MUFFIN: CALORIES: 110; FAT: 2.5 G; CHOLESTEROL: 0 MG; SODIUM: 145 MG;

PROTEIN: 3 G; CARBOHYDRATE: 21 G

# Applesauce-Oatmeal Muffins

*Liane F.*

MAKES 18 MUFFINS

A SNACK RECIPE given to me by Liane inspired these muffins, which are hearty, filling and practically fat-free. Serve with yogurt or a glass of skim milk.

1½ cups all-purpose flour
1 cup uncooked old-fashioned oatmeal
½ cup light or dark brown sugar
1¼ teaspoons baking powder
1 teaspoon baking soda
1 teaspoon ground cinnamon
½ teaspoon ground nutmeg
½ teaspoon salt
1 large egg
½ cup nonfat plain yogurt
¾ cup unsweetened applesauce
½ cup chopped pitted dates
½ cup skim milk

1. Preheat oven to 350 degrees F. Spray muffin pans with nonstick cooking spray or use paper cupcake liners. Set aside.

2. In a large mixing bowl, stir together flour, oatmeal, brown sugar, baking powder, baking soda, cinnamon, nutmeg and salt. Set aside.

3. In a medium bowl, whisk together egg, yogurt, applesauce, dates and milk.

4. Pour liquid ingredients over dry ingredients. Stir with a wooden spoon or a rubber spatula just until blended; do not overmix.

5. Spoon batter into prepared muffin pans, filling each cup about three-fourths full. Bake until muffins are lightly browned and a toothpick inserted in center comes out clean, about 20 minutes. Cool for 5 minutes in pans. Turn out and cool on wire racks before serving.

PER MUFFIN: CALORIES: 98; FAT: 0.5 G; CHOLESTEROL: 12 MG; SODIUM: 176 MG;

PROTEIN: 3 G; CARBOHYDRATE: 21 G

# Apricot-Orange Nut Bread

*Diane J.*

MAKES 1 LOAF, 12 SLICES

THIS DELECTABLE SWEET BREAD, made without added butter, margarine or oil, is wonderful with morning coffee or perfect for a fancy brunch. It gets even tastier after it sits for a day or two.

¾ cup dried apricots (about 4 ounces),
cut into ¼-inch pieces
2 cups all-purpose flour
⅓ cup pecan halves (about 1.3 ounces),
finely chopped
½ teaspoon baking powder
½ teaspoon salt
¼ teaspoon baking soda
1 large egg
1 cup granulated sugar
¾ cup orange juice
1 jar (4 ounces) pureed apricot baby food

1. Preheat oven to 350 degrees F, with a rack in center. Spray an 8½-x-4½-x-2½-inch loaf pan with nonstick cooking spray. Set aside.

2. **Microwave method:** Place dried apricots in a small microwavable bowl. Pour in enough water just to cover apricots. Microwave on high power for 2 minutes. Let stand for 10 minutes, or until you are ready to use them.

(**Stovetop method:** Bring 1½ cups water to a boil in a medium saucepan. Add dried apricots, remove from heat and let stand for 20 to 30 minutes, or until softened.)

3. Mix flour, pecans, baking powder, salt and baking soda in a large bowl until well blended. Set aside.

4. In a medium mixing bowl, with an electric mixer or a wire whisk, beat egg and sugar together until light in color. Add orange juice and pureed apricots. Mix well.

5. Drain apricots and add to flour mixture. With a wooden spoon or a rubber spatula, gently add liquid ingredients to dry ingredients, mixing until just moistened; do not overmix.

6. Pour into prepared loaf pan and bake for 55 to 60 minutes, or until a toothpick inserted in center comes out clean. Cool for 10 minutes in pan, then remove from pan and cool on a wire rack.

PER SLICE: CALORIES: 201; FAT: 3 G; CHOLESTEROL: 18 MG; SODIUM: 143 MG; PROTEIN: 3 G; CARBOHYDRATE: 41 G

# Light Rye Zucchini Bread

*Irene H.*

MAKES 1 LOAF, 12 SLICES

EVEN KIDS LIKE THIS unique quick bread made from cracker crumbs, oat bran, zucchini, spices and brown sugar. Rich-tasting and filling, it makes a quick, nutritious breakfast or snack. Have it with a glass of skim milk or a mug of low-fat latte. If you prefer a sweeter bread, use ⅔ cup brown sugar—I like it both ways.

8   Ryvita Light Rye Crisp Breads, crushed
    to very fine crumbs
8   Wasa Brod Wheat Crackers, crushed to
    very fine crumbs
1   cup oat bran
⅓-⅔ cup light or dark brown sugar
¼   cup nonfat dry milk powder
1   teaspoon baking powder
1   teaspoon ground cinnamon
½   teaspoon baking soda
½   teaspoon ground allspice
1   cup shredded zucchini
    (1 medium, about 6 ounces)
2   large eggs
⅓   cup water
3   tablespoons corn or safflower oil
1   teaspoon lemon juice

1. Preheat oven to 350 degrees F, with a rack in center. Spray an 8½-x-4½-x-2½-inch loaf pan with nonstick cooking spray and set aside.

2. In a large mixing bowl with a wooden spoon, stir together all dry ingredients. Set aside.

3. In a medium bowl, whisk together zucchini, eggs, water, oil and lemon juice. Pour liquid ingredients into dry ingredients and stir with a wooden spoon or a rubber spatula just until moistened.

4. Pour into loaf pan and bake for 30 to 35 minutes, or until a toothpick inserted in center comes out clean. Cool for 10 to 15 minutes in pan, then run a knife around edges of pan to loosen; remove from pan and cool on a wire rack before serving.

PER SLICE: CALORIES: 144; FAT: 5 G; CHOLESTEROL: 36 MG; SODIUM: 159 MG;

PROTEIN: 5 G; CARBOHYDRATE: 24 G

# Cornmeal Pancakes

*Diane J.*

MAKES ABOUT 10 PANCAKES

I F YOU LIKE CORN BREAD, you'll enjoy these light, golden pancakes. Top them with maple syrup or jam, with a light sprinkling of powdered sugar.

¾ cup all-purpose flour
½ cup yellow cornmeal
2 tablespoons granulated sugar
4 teaspoons baking powder
¾ teaspoon salt
2 large eggs
1 cup skim milk
1 tablespoon vegetable oil
1 teaspoon vanilla extract

1. In a large bowl, thoroughly mix flour, cornmeal, sugar, baking powder and salt. Set aside.

2. In a small bowl, whisk together eggs, milk, oil and vanilla. Pour liquid ingredients over dry ingredients. Whisk just until blended. (Don't worry if a few lumps remain; they'll work themselves out when cooking.)

3. Spray a large nonstick skillet or griddle with nonstick cooking spray. Heat over medium-high heat until hot enough to evaporate a drop of water immediately upon contact.

4. Spoon batter by ¼-cup measures onto hot skillet or griddle. Cook until evenly covered with bubbles, about 2 minutes. Using a spatula, carefully turn over and cook for 1 to 2 minutes more, until lightly browned. Repeat with remaining batter. (You may need to spray skillet or griddle with nonstick cooking spray between each batch. Lower heat to medium if pancakes are browning too quickly.) Keep pancakes warm in a low oven while you cook remaining batches.

PER PANCAKE: CALORIES: 103; FAT: 2.5 G; CHOLESTEROL: 43 MG; SODIUM: 382 MG;

PROTEIN: 4 G; CARBOHYDRATE: 16 G

# Whole Wheat Banana Pancakes

*K. W. H.*

KIDS AND GROWN-UPS ALIKE love these banana pancakes, which are great with maple syrup or jam. You can also roll them up fajita-style with a thin layer of peanut butter or a sprinkling of cinnamon and sugar.

|       |                                                              |
|-------|--------------------------------------------------------------|
| 1½    | cups whole wheat flour                                       |
| 1½    | cups all-purpose flour                                       |
| 2¼    | teaspoons baking powder                                      |
| 3     | large egg whites                                             |
| 1½    | cups skim milk                                               |
| 1     | teaspoon vanilla extract                                     |
| ¼     | teaspoon salt                                                |
| 1½    | cups mashed very ripe banana                                 |
|       | (about 3 medium or 17-18 ounces before peeling)              |
| 2     | teaspoons vegetable oil                                      |

1. In a small mixing bowl, stir together flours and baking powder until well blended. Set aside.

2. In a large mixing bowl, whisk together egg whites, milk, vanilla, salt, banana and oil. Pour liquid ingredients into dry ingredients and stir with a wooden spoon or a rubber spatula just until blended.

3. Spray a large nonstick skillet or griddle with nonstick cooking spray. Heat over medium-high heat until hot enough to evaporate a drop of water immediately upon contact.

4. Spoon batter by ¼-cup measures onto hot skillet or griddle. Cook until pancakes are slightly dry around edges and bubbles appear on top, about 2 minutes. Using a spatula, carefully turn over and cook for 1 to 2 minutes more, until lightly browned. Repeat with remaining batter. (You may need to spray skillet or griddle with nonstick cooking spray between each batch. Lower heat to medium if pancakes are browning too quickly.) Keep pancakes warm in a low oven while you cook remaining batches.

PER PANCAKE: CALORIES: 118; FAT: 1 G; CHOLESTEROL: 0 MG; SODIUM: 125 MG;

PROTEIN: 4 G; CARBOHYDRATE: 23 G

# Buttermilk-Spice Biscuits

*August J.*

MAKES 18 BISCUITS

THESE HEARTY FOUR-GRAIN DROP BISCUITS work well for dinner (with the lower spice level) or for breakfast (with the higher spice level). Either way, they're best served warm with a little honey, jam or diet margarine. You could also bake them with an added handful of raisins or some chopped apple.

|   |   |
|---|---|
| 2 | cups all-purpose flour |
| 1 | cup uncooked quick-cooking oatmeal |
| ½ | cup rye flour |
| ½ | cup yellow cornmeal |
| 1-2 | teaspoons ground cinnamon |
| 1-2 | teaspoons ground nutmeg |
| 1 | teaspoon baking powder |
| 1 | teaspoon baking soda |
| ½ | teaspoon ground ginger |
| ½ | teaspoon salt |
| 1½ | cups buttermilk |
| ¼ | cup vegetable oil |
| ¼ | cup honey |

1. Preheat oven to 400 degrees F, with a rack in center. Spray a cookie sheet with nonstick cooking spray. Set aside.

2. In a large mixing bowl, whisk together dry ingredients. Set aside.

3. In a small bowl, mix buttermilk, oil and honey. With a wooden spoon, gently stir buttermilk mixture into dry ingredients just until moistened.

4. Drop dough by ¼-cup measures onto cookie sheet and bake for 12 to 14 minutes, or until a toothpick inserted in center comes out clean. Serve warm. (Leftover biscuits should be cooled completely, then stored in a plastic bag or covered container.)

PER BISCUIT: CALORIES: 140; FAT: 4 G; CHOLESTEROL: 0 MG; SODIUM: 225 MG; PROTEIN: 3 G; CARBOHYDRATE: 23 G

# Golden Fruit Turnovers

*Jennie C.*

MAKES 8 TURNOVERS

THESE TURNOVERS make festive breakfast or brunch fare but can also serve as a low-fat dessert. (Jennie calls them "pielets.") For a special touch, drizzle each turnover with a glaze of powdered sugar mixed with a little skim milk.

FRUIT FILLING

1  cup chopped dried fruit (approximately 6 ounces), such as peaches, apricots or a mixture
1½  cups water
½  cup granulated sugar
1  teaspoon ground cinnamon

BISCUIT DOUGH

2  cups reduced-fat baking mix (such as Bisquick), plus some for dusting
1  tablespoon granulated sugar
¾  cup skim milk

1. Preheat oven to 350 degrees F, with a rack in center. Spray a cookie sheet with nonstick cooking spray. Set aside.

2. **To make fruit filling:** Place dried fruit and water in a medium saucepan. Bring to a boil over medium-high heat. Cover, reduce heat to low and simmer for about 30 minutes, or until fruit is soft. Remove from heat and mash with a fork until semi-smooth. (Some lumps should remain.) Stir in sugar and cinnamon. Cool in refrigerator for about 20 minutes.

3. **To make biscuit dough:** In a medium bowl, stir together baking mix and sugar. Add milk and blend with a fork until mixture forms a dough. Dust a work surface with extra baking mix, then turn dough out onto surface. Sprinkle with additional baking mix. Form dough into a ball. Roll or pat to ¼-inch thickness and cut eight 5-inch rounds with a cookie or tart cutter. Place rounds on prepared cookie sheet.

4. **To make turnovers:** Place about 2 tablespoons fruit filling just to left or right of center of each round. Fold one-half of dough over other half to enclose filling, forming a half moon. Crimp edges with fork.

5. Bake turnovers for 20 minutes, or until golden brown. Cool on a wire rack until you can handle them. Serve warm or at room temperature.

PER TURNOVER: CALORIES: 226; FAT: 2 G; CHOLESTEROL: 0 MG; SODIUM: 398 MG; PROTEIN: 4 G; CARBOHYDRATE: 49 G

# Breakfast Bars

*Lois A.*

MAKES 20 BARS

THE PERFECT RECIPE FOR BREAKFAST SKIPPERS: cereal, fruit and milk—all in a bar that you can make ahead and take with you as you race out the door in the morning.

| | |
|---|---|
| 1 | cup uncooked quick-cooking oatmeal |
| 1 | regular-sized shredded-wheat bar, crumbled |
| ½ | cup Grape-Nuts cereal |
| ½ | cup all-purpose flour |
| ¼ | cup light or dark brown sugar |
| 3 | teaspoons ground cinnamon |
| 2 | teaspoons ground nutmeg |
| 1½ | teaspoons baking soda |
| ½ | cup raisins (preferably golden raisins) |
| 4 | tablespoons (½ stick) melted margarine |
| 1 | can (14½ ounces) evaporated skim milk |
| 1 | cup unsweetened applesauce |
| 1 | teaspoon vanilla extract or ¼ teaspoon coconut extract |

1. Preheat oven to 350 degrees F, with a rack in center. Spray a 9-x-13-inch pan with nonstick cooking spray. Set aside.

2. In a large bowl, thoroughly combine dry ingredients, including raisins. Set aside.

3. In a small bowl, whisk together margarine, milk, applesauce and vanilla or coconut extract. Add to dry ingredients and mix with a wooden spoon or a rubber spatula just until combined. Pour evenly into prepared pan.

4. Bake for 25 to 30 minutes, or until a toothpick inserted in center comes out clean.

5. Cut into bars about 2¼ x 2½ inches. Serve warm or at room temperature. (To store, cool in pan, then tightly cover with foil.)

PER BAR: CALORIES: 105; FAT: 2.5 G; CHOLESTEROL: 0 MG; SODIUM: 210 MG;

PROTEIN: 3 G; CARBOHYDRATE: 17 G

# Kate's Granola

*Catherine C.*

MAKES ABOUT 16 SERVINGS, EACH ½ CUP

FILLED WITH HEALTHFUL GRAINS AND FIBER, this granola can be served with skim milk and fresh berries for breakfast or enjoyed dry as a snack.

4 cups uncooked quick-cooking oatmeal
1 cup bran flakes cereal
½ cup Bran Buds cereal
½ cup Grape-Nuts cereal
½ cup wheat germ
½ cup unsalted sunflower seeds
¼ cup light or dark brown sugar
½ teaspoon ground nutmeg
½ teaspoon ground cinnamon
¾ cup water
½ cup honey
1 cup dark or light raisins

1. Preheat oven to 300 degrees F, or for a crunchier cereal, 325 degrees. Spray a jellyroll pan with nonstick cooking spray.

2. In a large bowl, stir together oatmeal, bran flakes, Bran Buds, Grape-Nuts, wheat germ, sunflower seeds, brown sugar, nutmeg and cinnamon. Set aside.

3. In a small saucepan over medium heat, heat water and honey until well blended, stirring occasionally. Slowly add to cereal mixture, tossing to combine.

4. Spread cereal mixture across prepared jellyroll pan and bake for 50 to 60 minutes, stirring occasionally, until cereal is golden brown and of desired crunchiness. Remove from oven and add raisins. Cool, then store in an airtight container.

PER SERVING: CALORIES: 210; FAT: 4 G; CHOLESTEROL: 0 MG; SODIUM: 267 MG;

PROTEIN: 7 G; CARBOHYDRATE: 41 G

# Sandwiches and Soups

# Mock Egg Salad Sandwich

*Dorothy S.*

SERVES 2

I
F EGG SALAD used to be one of your favorite sandwiches but you're trying now to stay away from eggs (or even if you're not), this is a tasty alternative. It is simple to make and is best served on toasted bread.

½   cup (4-ounce carton) egg substitute, thawed
2   tablespoons sweet pickle relish
2   tablespoons finely chopped celery
2   tablespoons finely chopped green onion
    Salt and freshly ground black pepper to taste (optional)
4   slices whole wheat bread
1   tablespoon Dijon-style mustard
2   tablespoons nonfat mayonnaise
2   large lettuce leaves (optional)

1. Preheat oven to 375 degrees F. Spray a 10-inch ovenproof skillet or round baking pan with nonstick cooking spray. Pour in egg substitute and bake for 8 to 10 minutes, or until set.

2. Remove from oven and place egg on a plate. Cut in half to form 2 half-moon shapes. Spread a layer of relish on one-half of each half moon, then sprinkle with celery, green onion and salt and pepper, if desired. Fold plain halves over filling to enclose; set aside. (If desired, chill for 30 minutes.)

3. Spread bread with mustard and mayonnaise. Place each egg half on 1 slice of bread. Add lettuce. Top with remaining bread and serve.

PER SERVING: CALORIES: 215; FAT: 5 G; CHOLESTEROL: 1 MG; SODIUM: 732 MG; PROTEIN: 13 G; CARBOHYDRATE: 32 G

# Thai Salad Rolls

*Kelly S.*

MAKES 6 SALAD ROLLS

THIS SPICY COMBINATION of cellophane noodles, vegetables, cilantro, Chinese flavorings and peanut butter (of all things) in whole wheat tortillas tastes like a sesame-flavored vegetarian egg roll. In the original recipe, 60 percent of the calories came from fat; Kelly's rendition provides just 24 percent of calories from fat. (Cellophane noodles, sometimes called "bean threads," can be purchased, along with rice vinegar and hoisin sauce, in the Asian section of supermarkets.)

|   |   |
|---|---|
| 2 | ounces cellophane noodles |
| 1 | medium carrot, shredded (½ cup) |
| 1 | cup shredded cabbage |
| 1 | large celery stalk, chopped (¾ cup) |
| 1 | cup mung bean sprouts |
| ½ | cup chopped fresh cilantro |
| 3 | tablespoons rice vinegar |
| 2 | tablespoons soy sauce |
| 1 | tablespoon peanut butter |
| 1 | tablespoon hoisin sauce |
| 1½ | teaspoons Asian sesame oil |
| 6 | shakes Tabasco sauce |
| 1 | large garlic clove, minced |
| ½ | teaspoon ground ginger |
| 6 | whole wheat tortillas (8-inch size) |
| 12-18 | large spinach leaves |

1. Prepare cellophane noodles according to package directions or by soaking in boiling water for about 2 minutes, or until softened. Drain, rinse with cold water, then drain again. Cut noodles in half.

2. In a large mixing bowl, gently combine noodles, carrot, cabbage, celery, bean sprouts and cilantro. Set aside.

3. In a small bowl, whisk together vinegar, soy sauce, peanut butter, hoisin sauce, oil, Tabasco, garlic and ginger. (This can also be done in a blender.)

4. Pour sauce over noodle mixture, and toss well to coat. Refrigerate for 30 minutes to mellow flavors.

5. Warm tortillas in a microwave or, wrapped in foil, in a preheated 350-degree-F oven for about 10 minutes.

6. Lay several spinach leaves on top of each tortilla. Place one-sixth of salad mixture on top of spinach, distributing down center. Fold one side of tortilla over vegetables, then roll up to enclose. Serve immediately.

PER SALAD ROLL: CALORIES: 229; FAT: 6 G; CHOLESTEROL: 0 MG; SODIUM: 660 MG; PROTEIN: 6 G; CARBOHYDRATE: 39 G

# Hawaiian Pizza Pockets

*Dorothy S.*

MAKES 4 SANDWICH HALVES

T HIS SIMPLE LOW-FAT PIZZA combination enlivened with pineapple, green pepper and mushrooms is wonderful for lunch at the office, where you can "zap" the pockets in a microwave.

2 pita pocket breads (each 6 inches in diameter), cut in half
2 ounces sliced Canadian bacon (4 slices)
¼ cup pizza sauce or reduced-fat spaghetti sauce
½ cup chopped green bell pepper (1 small)
½ cup chopped fresh mushrooms (about 2 ounces)
¼ cup shredded part-skim mozzarella cheese (1 ounce)
2 rings canned juice-packed pineapple, cut in half

1. Preheat oven to 350 degrees F. Open each pita bread half to form a pocket. Inside each pocket lay 1 slice Canadian bacon. Top with 1 tablespoon pizza or spaghetti sauce, 2 tablespoons green pepper, 2 tablespoons mushrooms, 1 tablespoon mozzarella and one-half of a pineapple ring.

2. Set sandwich pockets upright, open sides facing upward, in a 9-x-5-inch loaf pan, and cover tightly with aluminum foil. Bake for 7 to 10 minutes, or until cheese is melted and sandwich is heated through. (You can also warm pockets in a microwave for about 20 seconds on high power.) Serve hot.

PER HALF: CALORIES: 156; FAT: 3 G; CHOLESTEROL: 11 MG; SODIUM: 462 MG; PROTEIN: 8 G; CARBOHYDRATE: 25 G

# Chicken Wild Rice Soup

*JoAnna M. Lund*

SERVES 4

JoANNA NOTES, "This is so thick and creamy that you are going to swear it's loaded with fat. But it's not!" To save time when making it, she suggests buying already cooked chicken at the deli. Serve with fresh vegetables and dip and some warm rye or pumpernickel bread. This was adapted from a recipe in JoAnna Lund's *Healthy Exchanges Food Newsletter.*

4   cups defatted chicken broth
1   small onion, chopped (about ⅓ cup)
2   medium carrots, shredded (about 1 cup)
2   medium celery stalks, sliced (about 1 cup)
½   cup uncooked instant long-grain and wild rice mix
1   cup diced cooked skinless chicken breast
    (about 6 ounces)
1   can (10¾ ounces) Campbell's Healthy Request
    Cream of Mushroom Soup

1. In a large saucepan, combine broth, onion, carrots, celery and rice. Bring to a boil. Lower heat to medium and add chicken. Cover and continue cooking until vegetables are tender and rice is done, 10 to 12 minutes.

2. Stir in mushroom soup. Serve immediately.

PER SERVING: CALORIES: 206; FAT: 4 G; CHOLESTEROL: 33 MG; SODIUM: 1,162 MG; PROTEIN: 18 G; CARBOHYDRATE: 22 G

# Basil Beef Dumpling Soup

*Gaylord J.*

SERVES 6 TO 8

WITH ITS SUBSTANTIAL BROTH filled with meat and vegetables, this satisfying soup is a cross between a soup and a stew. If all the dumplings are gone after the first time you serve it, you can make another batch and add more before serving it again.

SOUP

1 pound round steak, trimmed and
  cut into bite-sized cubes
1 package onion soup mix
6 cups water
3 cups defatted beef broth
4 medium celery stalks, sliced (about 2 cups)
2 medium carrots, shredded (about 1 cup)
1 large carrot, cut into coins (about 1 cup)
1 medium red bell pepper, chopped (about 1 cup)
1 large onion, chopped (about 1 cup)
1 large ripe or green tomato, chopped (about 1 cup)

DUMPLINGS

1 cup reduced-fat baking mix (such as Bisquick)
3 tablespoons shredded Parmesan cheese
1 tablespoon dried basil
6 tablespoons skim milk

1. **To make soup:** Spray a large pot with nonstick cooking spray. Add steak and soup mix. Mix and brown for about 5 minutes over medium-high heat.

2. Stir in water, broth, celery, sliced and shredded carrots, red pepper, onion and tomato. Bring to a boil, stirring occasionally. Reduce heat to low, partially cover, and simmer for 1½ to 2 hours, or until beef is tender.

3. **To make dumplings:** About 25 minutes before soup is done, combine baking mix, Parmesan and basil in a small bowl. Stir in milk with a fork until mixture is moistened. When beef is tender, drop dumpling dough into broth by rounded teaspoonfuls, one at a time. (Do not stir soup.) Over medium heat, cook, uncovered, for 10 minutes. Cover and cook for 10 minutes more, or until cooked through. Serve immediately.

PER SERVING: CALORIES: 189; FAT: 4 G; CHOLESTEROL: 31 MG; SODIUM: 1,236 MG;

PROTEIN: 16 G; CARBOHYDRATE: 22 G

# Heartland Corn Chowder

*JoAnna M. Lund*

SERVES 4

H AM, CORN, CHOPPED POTATO and mushrooms give a flavorful, chunky texture to this creamy, cheesy soup. JoAnna describes it as "rib-sticking." It makes a complete meal with some Italian bread and a tossed salad. The recipe was adapted from one in JoAnna Lund's *Healthy Exchanges Food Newsletter*.

1 small-to-medium onion, chopped (about ½ cup)
1 cup diced extra-lean cooked ham (about 5 ounces)
2 cups frozen corn kernels
1 large potato, unpeeled, cooked and diced
   (about 8 ounces or 1 heaping cup)
½ cup canned sliced mushrooms
   (2½-ounce jar), drained
1 can (10¾ ounces) Campbell's
   Healthy Request Cream of Mushroom Soup
1⅓ cups skim milk
¾ cup shredded reduced-fat Cheddar cheese
   (about 3 ounces)
1 teaspoon prepared mustard
1 teaspoon Sprinkle Sweet or Sugar Twin
1 teaspoon dried parsley flakes
¼ teaspoon freshly ground black pepper

1. In a large saucepan sprayed with butter-flavored cooking spray, sauté onion and ham over medium-high heat, stirring often, until onion is tender, about 5 minutes.

2. Stir in corn, potato, mushrooms, soup and milk. Cover and simmer, stirring occasionally, for 5 to 7 minutes, or until hot.

3. Reduce heat to low and stir in cheese, mustard, sweetener, parsley and pepper. Simmer for another 5 to 7 minutes to blend flavors and melt cheese, stirring occasionally. Serve immediately.

PER SERVING: CALORIES: 304; FAT: 7 G; CHOLESTEROL: 34 MG; SODIUM: 1,040 MG; PROTEIN: 20 G; CARBOHYDRATE: 42 G

# Thick and Chunky Minestrone

*Joy C.*

SERVES 8 TO 10

O N A COLD WINTER NIGHT, nothing makes you feel better than a steaming one-pot meal of tomato, beef, vegetables and noodles. The list of ingredients is long, but the recipe is easy!

½   pound extra-lean ground beef
1   large onion, chopped (about 1 cup)
2   large garlic cloves, minced
1   small green bell pepper, chopped (about ½ cup)
6   cups defatted reduced-sodium beef broth
2   cups V-8 juice
2   cups water
1   can (15 ounces) Italian-style stewed tomatoes, with juice
1   large carrot, sliced (about 1 cup)
⅓   cup barley
1   tablespoon dried basil
1   bay leaf
¼   pound cabbage, chopped (about 1½ cups)
1   can (15 ounces) kidney beans, undrained
1   medium zucchini (6 ounces), sliced
1   cup dried rotini
2   tablespoons lemon juice

1. Brown ground beef in a large Dutch oven over medium-high heat. Drain fat and return to medium heat. Add onion, garlic and green pepper. Cook, uncovered, stirring often, until onion becomes translucent but not brown, 5 to 7 minutes.

2. Add broth, V-8 juice, water, tomatoes, carrot, barley, basil and bay leaf. Cover and simmer over medium heat for 25 to 30 minutes, or until barley is almost tender.

3. Stir in cabbage, kidney beans, zucchini, rotini and lemon juice. Simmer, uncovered, for 15 to 18 minutes, or until rotini is tender. Remove bay leaf and serve.

PER SERVING: CALORIES: 181; FAT: 2.5 G; CHOLESTEROL: 14 MG; SODIUM: 825 MG;

PROTEIN: 12 G; CARBOHYDRATE: 28 G

# Luscious Black Bean Soup

*Don Mauer*

SERVES 6 TO 8

QUICK AND COLORFUL, this soup is a great centerpiece for a cozy winter supper—serve with a tossed salad and warm bagels. A dollop of nonfat sour cream on each serving and a spoonful of salsa or a sprinkling of snipped chives make tasty, guiltless additions. This recipe was adapted from one in Don Mauer's *Lean and Lovin' It* (Chapters Publishing).

2  teaspoons olive oil
2  large onions, chopped
1  large green bell pepper, chopped
1  large red bell pepper, chopped
½  cup chopped fresh cilantro leaves
1  teaspoon dried oregano leaves
1  bay leaf
1  cup defatted chicken broth
3  cans (15 ounces each) black beans, undrained (salted or unsalted)
4  low-fat hot dogs (no more than 2 grams fat each), thinly sliced
¼  cup apple cider vinegar
1  teaspoon granulated sugar

1. In a large soup kettle or Dutch oven, heat oil over medium-high heat. When oil is hot, add onions and peppers. Sauté, stirring, for 4 to 5 minutes, until vegetables are softened but not browned.

2. Add cilantro, oregano and bay leaf and sauté for 1 minute more. Stir in broth, beans with their liquid and hot dogs, and bring to a boil, stirring frequently. Immediately reduce heat and simmer, covered, for 5 minutes.

3. Remove soup from heat, and stir in vinegar and sugar. Remove bay leaf before serving. Serve immediately.

PER SERVING: CALORIES: 255; FAT: 3 G; CHOLESTEROL: 8 MG; SODIUM: 1,030 MG; PROTEIN: 17 G; CARBOHYDRATE: 42 G

# Chicken Egg Drop Soup

*Diane J.*

SERVES 8 AS AN APPETIZER OR 4 AS A MEAL

Diane's light and easy broth-based soup is terrific for lunch—try it with a Chinese cabbage salad with low-fat dressing. This also makes a great first course when serving a Chinese-style dish, such as Vegetable Tofu Stir-Fry (page 262) or Moo Goo Gai Pan (page 216). My kids love this soup so much that they asked for thirds one night!

5 cups defatted chicken broth
½ teaspoon granulated sugar
  Generous grating black pepper
¼ cup cold water
3 tablespoons cornstarch
2 large eggs, beaten with a whisk
1 cup diced cooked skinless chicken breast
  (about 6 ounces)
1 cup chopped green onions (about 2 bunches)

1. Pour broth into a large saucepan and stir in sugar and pepper. Bring to a boil over medium-high heat.

2. Meanwhile, in a small bowl, whisk cold water slowly into cornstarch until a smooth paste forms. When broth comes to a boil, whisk in cornstarch mixture, return to a boil and cook for 1 minute, stirring constantly, until mixture is slightly thickened and translucent.

3. Remove from heat, and slowly whisk in eggs, a small amount at a time, separating egg into thin strands.

4. Over low heat, stir in chicken and green onions. Cover and simmer for 1 to 2 minutes, or until chicken is heated through. Serve immediately.

PER APPETIZER SERVING: CALORIES: 88; FAT: 2.5 G; CHOLESTEROL: 68 MG; SODIUM: 516 MG; PROTEIN: 10 G; CARBOHYDRATE: 5 G

# Snacks, Appetizers and Dips

# Blue Cheese Deviled Eggs

*Ann F.*

MAKES 12 HALVES

A BLUE CHEESE-MUSTARD COMBINATION puts a new spin on deviled eggs—and they're low in fat. You can also add sweet pickle relish or finely chopped green onions or celery to the yolk mixture.

6   hard-cooked eggs, cooled, peeled and cut in half
3   tablespoons fat-free blue cheese dressing
2   teaspoons mild yellow (American-style) mustard
    Paprika for sprinkling on top

1. Scoop out yolks into a small bowl. Mash finely with a fork.

2. Mix dressing and mustard into mashed yolks. Stuff egg white halves with yolk mixture. Sprinkle with paprika. Cover and refrigerate until ready to serve. Serve cold.

PER HALF: CALORIES: 44; FAT: 3 G; CHOLESTEROL: 106 MG; SODIUM: 42 MG; PROTEIN: 3 G; CARBOHYDRATE: 1 G

# Spinach Balls

*Diane J.*

MAKES APPROXIMATELY 20 BALLS

OR A PARTY APPETIZER or everyday snacking, these festive balls of spinach and cheese hit the spot. They're especially appealing for the do-ahead cook, because you can mix, shape and freeze them up to 2 weeks before baking.

  1   package (10 ounces) frozen chopped spinach,
      thawed and well drained
 ¾   cup shredded reduced-fat Swiss or
      Colby cheese (3 ounces)
 ¼   cup nonfat salad dressing (such as Miracle Whip)
 ¼   cup unseasoned bread crumbs
  1   small onion, grated (about ¼ cup)
  1   large egg, slightly beaten
  2   tablespoons shredded Parmesan cheese
  1   tablespoon Dijon-style mustard

1. Preheat oven to 325 degrees F. Spray a cookie sheet with nonstick cooking spray and set aside.

2. In a medium bowl, with a fork, mix all ingredients. Shape into 1-inch balls and place on cookie sheet. (At this point, you can place the balls in an airtight container and freeze.)

3. Bake for approximately 15 to 20 minutes, or until golden brown around edges and piping hot in centers. Serve hot.

PER 2-BALL SERVING: CALORIES: 60; FAT: 2.5 G; CHOLESTEROL: 27 MG; SODIUM: 170 MG; PROTEIN: 4 G; CARBOHYDRATE: 6G

# Cilantro-Veggie Fajitas

*Stan J.*

MAKES 4 FAJITAS

THE TORTILLAS ARE SPREAD with nonfat cream cheese and rolled up around a colorful combination of steamed red and green onions, zucchini, carrots, mushrooms and cilantro. Serve warm or cold, whole or cut into 1-inch slices as an appetizer. If desired, top with taco sauce or salsa.

½ cup chopped green onions (approximately 1 bunch)
1 medium zucchini (6-7 ounces), quartered and thinly sliced
1 large carrot, thinly sliced (about ¾ cup)
4 ounces fresh mushrooms, cleaned and chopped (about 1 cup)
1 small red onion, chopped (about ⅓ cup)
4 tablespoons chopped fresh cilantro
4 soft flour tortillas (9-to-10-inch diameter), warmed
4 tablespoons nonfat cream cheese
4 tablespoons shredded Parmesan cheese (about 1 ounce)

1. Spray a large nonstick skillet with nonstick cooking spray. Add green onions, zucchini, carrot, mushrooms, red onion and cilantro, and sauté over medium-high heat until heated through and just starting to wilt, 3 to 5 minutes. Cover and set aside.

2. On each warm tortilla, spread 1 tablespoon cream cheese. Divide vegetables evenly among tortillas. Sprinkle each with 1 tablespoon Parmesan and roll up. Serve immediately or refrigerate and serve cold.

PER FAJITA: CALORIES: 217; FAT: 5 G; CHOLESTEROL: 6 MG; SODIUM: 414 MG; PROTEIN: 11 G; CARBOHYDRATE: 34 G

# Mexican Bean Roll-Up

## *K. W. H.*

SERVES 8 GENEROUSLY

TAKE A PIZZA CRUST, top it with Mexican fixings and sun-dried tomatoes, then roll it into a jellyroll, slice it into pinwheels, and you've got a tasty appetizer. It also makes a great main course, presented unsliced on a large serving dish, surrounded by shredded lettuce and bowls of salsa, black olives and low-fat shredded cheese. (If spicy food isn't your thing, leave out the jalapeños.)

| | |
|---|---|
| 1 | ounce (about ⅓ cup) sun-dried tomatoes |
| 1 | refrigerated tube pizza crust (about 10 ounces) |
| 1 | can (16 ounces) fat-free refried beans |
| ½ | cup nonfat sour cream |
| 1 | large onion, chopped (about 1 cup) |
| 1 | medium green bell pepper, chopped (about 1 cup) |
| ⅓-½ | cup sliced jalapeño peppers |

1. Cover sun-dried tomatoes with boiling water and soak for 10 to 15 minutes, or until softened. Drain; coarsely chop.

2. Meanwhile, preheat oven to 425 degrees F. Spray a jellyroll pan with nonstick cooking spray. Spread pizza dough to edges of pan and bake for 6 minutes, or until crust is set and lightly browned. Remove from oven and reduce heat to 350 degrees.

3. Immediately turn pan upside down, transferring crust to a towel-covered cooling rack. Carefully roll up crust in a towel so it will be easier to roll later. Cool, still wrapped in towel.

SNACKS, APPETIZERS AND DIPS

4. In a small bowl, with a fork, mix beans and sun-dried tomatoes. Unroll crust and spread top with bean-tomato mixture. On top of beans and in separate layers, evenly distribute sour cream, onion, green pepper and jalapeños. Carefully roll up and place, seam side down, on jellyroll pan.

5. Bake for 15 minutes, or until golden brown. Slice into 8 pinwheels, and serve.

PER PINWHEEL: CALORIES: 194; FAT: 2 G; CHOLESTEROL: 0 MG; SODIUM: 635 MG;

PROTEIN: 9 G; CARBOHYDRATE: 36 G

# Creamy Dill Dip

*Paul R.*

MAKES ABOUT 2 CUPS OR 8 SERVINGS, EACH ¼ CUP

ONFAT SOUR CREAM and mayonnaise team up with dill, onion and seasonings in a creamy dip that's great with vegetables, crisp crackers or baked tortilla chips. It keeps in the refrigerator for weeks and also makes a flavorful binder for salmon or tuna salad. To turn it into a salad dressing, thin it with some buttermilk. (Beaumonde Seasoning, a blend of salt, sugar, onion and celery seed, is sold under the Spice Islands label.)

1   cup nonfat sour cream
1   cup nonfat mayonnaise
2   tablespoons dried parsley flakes
2   tablespoons dried dill weed
1   tablespoon minced onion
1   tablespoon Beaumonde Seasoning

1. In a medium bowl, whisk together sour cream and mayonnaise. Add remaining ingredients and mix well.

2. Cover and refrigerate for several hours to blend flavors. Serve cold.

PER SERVING: CALORIES: 55; FAT: 0 G; CHOLESTEROL: 0 MG; SODIUM: 303 MG;

PROTEIN: 2 G; CARBOHYDRATE: 10 G

# Chili Bean Dip

*Kay D.*

MAKES ABOUT 1½ CUPS OR 6 SERVINGS, EACH ¼ CUP

ERVE THIS DIP with reduced-fat crackers or chips and raw vegetables. It can also substitute for refried beans. Spread the dip on a tortilla and top with lettuce, salsa, low-fat cheese and a few black olives.

1   can (15 ounces) kidney beans, drained
1   small onion, chopped (about ⅓ cup)
2   tablespoons chili sauce
1   tablespoon apple cider vinegar
¾   teaspoon chili powder
⅛   teaspoon ground cumin
    Optional: ½ cup shredded reduced-fat Cheddar,
    Colby or Monterey Jack cheese (2 ounces)

1. Place beans, onion, chili sauce, vinegar, chili powder and cumin in a food processor fitted with the metal blade and pulse until smooth. (Mixture can also be mashed with a fork.)

2. If using cheese, place dip in a microwavable bowl and top with shredded cheese. Microwave on high power until cheese melts and center is warm, 1 to 2 minutes. (Or warm in an ovenproof bowl in a preheated 350-degree-F oven for 15 minutes.) Serve immediately.

PER SERVING: CALORIES: 66; FAT: 0 G; CHOLESTEROL: 0 MG; SODIUM: 251 MG;

PROTEIN: 4 G; CARBOHYDRATE: 12 G

# South-of-the-Border Salsa

*Keith Van Gasken*

MAKES ABOUT 2 CUPS OR 8 SERVINGS, EACH ¼ CUP

THIS HANDY SALSA doesn't rely on garden-grown tomatoes. It's terrific for low-fat tortilla chips as well as fresh vegetables.

| | |
|--|--|
| 1 | can (14 ounces) crushed tomatoes (about 1½ cups) |
| ½ | cup chopped fresh cilantro leaves |
| 1 | small red onion, finely chopped (¼-⅓ cup) |
| 1 | serrano chili pepper, seeded and finely chopped (use more if you like hotter salsa) |
| ½ | teaspoon salt |
| 3 | tablespoons lime juice, plus more to taste |

In a small bowl, mix all ingredients. Let salsa sit for about 1 hour to blend flavors. If desired, add more chili pepper and lime juice. If salsa is too watery, drain off a little juice before serving.

PER SERVING: CALORIES: 19; FAT: 0 G; CHOLESTEROL: 0 MG; SODIUM: 216 MG; PROTEIN: 1 G; CARBOHYDRATE: 4 G

# Pepper-Onion Mayonnaise Dip

*K. W. H.*

MAKES ABOUT 1¼ CUPS OR 10 SERVINGS,
EACH 2 TABLESPOONS

THIS SAVORY FAT-FREE MAYONNAISE SUBSTITUTE is also good as a vegetable dip, in sandwiches and in pasta, potato, chicken or tuna salads. It can be thinned with a little buttermilk and turned into dressing for fresh salad greens.

| | |
|---|---|
| 1 | cup nonfat mayonnaise |
| 1 | large garlic clove, minced |
| 1 | tablespoon chopped fresh parsley |
| 1 | tablespoon chopped green bell pepper |
| 1 | tablespoon finely chopped onion |
| 1 | tablespoon chopped pimiento |
| 2 | teaspoons lemon juice |
| ⅛ | teaspoon ground paprika |
| | Generous grating black pepper |

In a small mixing bowl, with a wire whisk, thoroughly combine all ingredients. Refrigerate for several hours to blend flavors. Serve cold.

PER SERVING: CALORIES: 18; FAT: 0 G; CHOLESTEROL: 0 MG; SODIUM: 209 MG; PROTEIN: 0 G; CARBOHYDRATE: 4 G

# Main Dishes

## CHICKEN

## BEEF AND PORK

## SEAFOOD

# PASTA AND PIZZAS

# MEXICAN DISHES

# VEGETARIAN MAIN DISHES

# Sesame-Soy Chicken with Vegetables

*Molly A.*

SERVES 4

I THINK OF THIS DISH as a "microwave" stir-fry, except you don't have to stir it! (It can also be prepared in the oven.) The chicken is first marinated in soy sauce, then coated with Wasa Brod crumbs, which hold in moisture. No oil is needed. Serve with brown or white rice and sliced tomatoes.

16-18 ounces boneless, skinless chicken breast halves
(about 4), cut into 1-x-3-inch strips if microwaving,
left whole if cooking in oven

2 tablespoons soy sauce
Generous grating black pepper

1 small onion, sliced

1 small green bell pepper, chopped (about ½ cup)

1 small red bell pepper, chopped (about ½ cup)

1 cup sliced fresh mushrooms (about 4 ounces)

4 Wasa Brod crackers, your favorite flavor
(Sesame Rye works well), finely crushed

1 tablespoon toasted sesame seeds

1. Spray a 1½-quart microwavable or ovenproof casserole dish with nonstick cooking spray. If using oven, preheat to 375 degrees F.

2. Place chicken in casserole. Toss with soy sauce and pepper. Cover with plastic wrap and marinate in refrigerator for 15 minutes.

3. In a small bowl, mix onion, green and red peppers and mushrooms. Set aside.

4. Put cracker crumbs and sesame seeds in a large plastic bag. Place chicken in bag, several pieces or 1 breast at a time, and shake to coat well. Return chicken to casserole (leaving any marinade in bottom), and top with remaining crumbs.

5. **Microwave method**: Cover casserole with plastic wrap and puncture with several holes to allow steam to escape. Microwave on high power for 5 minutes. Rotate casserole. Add reserved vegetables and microwave for 5 minutes more. Cut into chicken to see if juices run clear. If chicken needs more cooking, microwave for 1-minute intervals until juices run clear and chicken pieces are no longer pink in center. (Don't overcook.)

**Oven method:** Add reserved vegetables to casserole and cover with foil. Bake for 20 minutes. Uncover and bake for 15 minutes more, or until juices run clear when you cut into thickest piece of chicken.

6. Serve immediately, piping hot.

PER SERVING: CALORIES: 245; FAT: 5 G; CHOLESTEROL: 82 MG; SODIUM: 695 MG; PROTEIN: 33 G; CARBOHYDRATE: 17 G

# Oven-Fried Chicken

*Don Mauer*

SERVES 6

ODAY WHEN DON MAUER craves the taste of fried chicken, once a regular part of his diet, he makes the following recipe, which is crumbly and loaded with lemony, garlicky flavor.

3   large garlic cloves, minced
1   teaspoon olive oil
1   cup unseasoned bread crumbs
2   tablespoons yellow cornmeal
1   tablespoon grated lemon rind
½   teaspoon salt
    Generous grating black pepper
¼   cup Dijon-style mustard
2   tablespoons water
1   rounded tablespoon honey
6   boneless, skinless chicken breast halves
    (about 1½ pounds)

1. Preheat oven to 425 degrees F, with a rack in center. Spray a rack set in a shallow baking pan with nonstick cooking spray. Set aside.

2. Combine garlic and oil in a small nonstick skillet. Sauté garlic over medium heat until slightly softened; do not brown. In a small bowl, combine garlic with bread crumbs, cornmeal, lemon rind, salt and pepper; mixture should be fine and uniform. Transfer to a shallow dish. Set aside.

3. In a shallow soup bowl, stir together mustard, water and honey.

4. Piece by piece, coat each breast with mustard mixture, then crumb mixture, turning several times and pressing crumbs into surfaces. As each piece is complete, place on prepared rack. Sprinkle lightly with 2 tablespoons remaining crumbs.

5. Bake for 20 minutes, or until chicken is crisp and juices run clear when it is cut in the middle. Serve immediately.

Per serving: calories: 235; fat: 5 g; cholesterol: 77 mg; sodium: 421 mg; protein: 31 g; carbohydrate: 15 g

# Chicken Piccata

*Patricia D.*

SERVES 4

L EMON, GARLIC, GREEN ONION AND CAPERS enliven boneless chicken breasts, which are sautéed and topped with lemon slices. Serve with seasoned rice, peas and Polynesian Carrot Salad (page 274).

4  boneless, skinless chicken breast halves
    (16-18 ounces total)
1  teaspoon Mrs. Dash Seasoning
1  teaspoon lemon pepper
1  tablespoon margarine or butter
1  medium onion, chopped (about ⅔ cup)
5  green onions (1 bunch), sliced with green parts
2  large garlic cloves, minced
⅓  cup capers, drained
¼  cup chopped fresh parsley
4  lemon slices, about ¼ inch thick, peeled
1  cup water

1. Sprinkle chicken breasts with Mrs. Dash Seasoning and lemon pepper. Spray a large nonstick skillet with nonstick cooking spray. Add chicken breasts and brown over medium-high heat for 5 to 7 minutes on each side. Remove chicken to a platter, cover, and set aside.

2. In same skillet, melt margarine or butter over medium heat. Add onion, green onions, garlic, capers, parsley and lemon slices. Sauté for 2 to 3 minutes, or until onion is translucent but not brown. Add chicken and water, and simmer, uncovered, for 10 minutes, or until juices run clear when a cut is made in center of chicken. Serve hot.

PER SERVING: CALORIES: 205; FAT: 6 G; CHOLESTEROL: 82 MG; SODIUM: 245 MG; PROTEIN: 31 G; CARBOHYDRATE: 5 G

# Middle Eastern Chicken

*Sam Eukel*

SERVES 4

A HINT OF CINNAMON AND ALLSPICE adds panache to this simple tomato-based dish. Serve over couscous or on a bed of rice. This was adapted from a recipe in Sam Eukel's *Sensibly Thin: Low-Fat Living and Cooking, Volume II.*

1 pound boneless, skinless chicken breasts
1 can (14½ ounces) diced tomatoes, with juice
2¼ cups defatted reduced-sodium chicken broth
½ package onion soup mix (about 2 tablespoons)
2 tablespoons tomato paste
1 can (14 ounces) artichoke hearts, drained and quartered (about 1 cup)
½ cup sliced black olives (2 ounces)
¼ teaspoon ground allspice
¼ teaspoon ground cinnamon

1. Cut chicken breasts into ½-x-1-inch pieces. Spray a large nonstick skillet with nonstick cooking spray, add chicken and sauté over medium-high heat for 2 to 3 minutes, or until browned.

2. Stir in tomatoes, broth, soup mix and tomato paste. Bring to a boil, reduce heat to low and simmer, uncovered, for 20 minutes.

3. Add artichokes, olives, allspice and cinnamon. Stir and simmer, uncovered, for another 5 minutes, or until no trace of pink remains in center of chicken. Serve hot.

PER SERVING: CALORIES: 238; FAT: 6 G; CHOLESTEROL: 70 MG; SODIUM: 1,250 MG; PROTEIN: 32 G; CARBOHYDRATE: 15 G

# Moo Goo Gai Pan

*Keith Van Gasken*

SERVES 4 GENEROUSLY

THIS SLIMMED-DOWN VERSION of my Chinese-restaurant favorite contains just a teaspoon of oil. Serve over a bed of hot, steamed rice, and you've got a complete meal. But for company, you might want to start with Chicken Egg Drop Soup (page 196).

5   dried Chinese black mushrooms
12  ounces boneless, skinless chicken breasts,
    cut into ½-x-2-inch strips
1   cup defatted chicken broth
1   can (8 ounces) sliced water chestnuts, drained
1   can (8 ounces) bamboo shoots, drained
1   can (4½ ounces) button mushrooms, drained
1   package (6 ounces) frozen snow pea pods
1   large garlic clove, minced
1   tablespoon oyster sauce
2   teaspoons soy sauce
1   teaspoon Asian sesame oil
2   tablespoons cornstarch

1. Soak black mushrooms in hot water to cover for 20 minutes, or until softened. Drain, discard stems, slice, and set aside.

2. Spray a wok or a large nonstick skillet with nonstick cooking spray. Over medium-high heat, sauté chicken for 5 to 6 minutes, or until no trace of pink remains. Remove and set aside.

3. Add ½ cup broth, water chestnuts, bamboo shoots, black and button mushrooms, snow peas, garlic, oyster sauce, soy sauce and sesame oil to wok or skillet. Stir frequently and gently, heating just until snow peas separate.

4. Meanwhile, in a small bowl, mix remaining ½ cup broth into corn-starch until no lumps remain. Add to vegetable mixture along with chicken. Stir gently and cook until sauce thickens, 3 to 5 minutes. Remove from heat and serve immediately.

PER SERVING: CALORIES: 222; FAT: 4 G; CHOLESTEROL: 58 MG; SODIUM: 365 MG;

PROTEIN: 25 G; CARBOHYDRATE: 18 G

# Crêpes with Chicken and Mushroom Filling

*Diane J.*

MAKES 12 CRÊPES; ENOUGH FILLING FOR 6 CRÊPES

W E AGREE WITH DIANE'S EXCLAMATION about her crêpes stuffed with a creamy chicken, mushroom and herb filling: "They are to die for!" She adds, "My grandkids love them." Accompany with a spinach salad and fresh cantaloupe or watermelon wedges. Incidentally, the unstuffed crêpes keep well, refrigerated in a plastic bag, so you can make them ahead. (This recipe makes some extra crêpes, which you can use for a simple yet elegant dessert—fill with jam or preserves and top with powdered sugar.) Note that the batter has to rest for at least 2 hours before cooking to allow the flour particles to absorb water, producing a tender, light and thin crêpe.

CRÊPES

½ cup cold water
½ cup skim milk
3 large eggs
1 tablespoon vegetable oil
1 cup all-purpose flour
1 teaspoon baking powder
¼ teaspoon salt

FILLING

2 tablespoons dry white wine
3 cups sliced fresh mushrooms (about 10 ounces)
1 tablespoon vegetable oil
3 tablespoons all-purpose flour
2 cups skim milk
⅓ cup chopped fresh chives
2 medium garlic cloves, minced
3 tablespoons chopped onion
1 teaspoon Molly McButter Butter Sprinkles
1 teaspoon Molly McButter Cheese Sprinkles

¼    teaspoon lemon pepper
¼    teaspoon dried thyme
2    boneless, skinless chicken breast halves
      (4-5 ounces each), cooked and cut into ½-inch cubes
2    tablespoons shredded Parmesan cheese

1. **To make crêpes**: In a medium bowl, whisk together water, milk, eggs and oil. Set aside.

2. In a small bowl, thoroughly combine flour, baking powder and salt. Whisk dry ingredients into liquid ingredients until well blended. Cover and refrigerate for at least 2 hours or overnight.

3. Heat a 6- or 7-inch crêpe pan or nonstick skillet sprayed with nonstick cooking spray over medium heat until a drop of water dances on the surface. Pour in a scant ¼ cup batter, tilting quickly to spread batter. Cook for 30 to 40 seconds, or until bottom is lightly browned. Turn with a rubber spatula and brown other side.

4. Tip crêpe out onto wax paper. Keep crêpes covered with a damp cloth so they don't dry out. Repeat until all batter is used. If not serving immediately, cool crêpes, stack and wrap well before refrigerating or freezing.

5. **To make filling**: Heat a large nonstick skillet over medium-high heat for about 2 minutes. Pour in wine and mushrooms, and sauté for 2 to 3 minutes, or until mushrooms begin to soften. Pour into a small bowl; set aside. Reduce heat to medium.

6. Add oil to skillet and stir in flour. Mixture will be dry. Using a wire whisk, slowly add milk to flour mixture, stirring constantly until mixture thickens. Stir in chives, garlic, onion, sprinkles, lemon pepper and thyme. Simmer for 1 minute to blend flavors.

7. Pour 1 cup sauce into a small bowl; set aside. Stir mushroom mixture and chicken into remaining sauce. Simmer for 3 to 5 minutes, or until heated through.

8. Meanwhile, preheat boiler and spray an ovenproof 8-x-11-inch baking dish with nonstick cooking spray. Set aside.

9. **To assemble crêpes:** Place a crêpe on a large plate. Place one-sixth of filling in center of crêpe and evenly distribute it down middle. Flip one side over filling and roll up crêpe. Place seam side down in prepared baking dish. Repeat with remaining 5 crêpes. Pour reserved 1 cup sauce over stuffed crêpes and sprinkle with Parmesan.

10. Place under broiler, 2 to 3 inches from heat, until sauce bubbles and is lightly browned, about 1 minute. (Watch closely.)

**To prepare ahead:** Refrigerate crêpes and sauce for filling and topping in separate containers. When ready to serve, assemble as detailed above. Bake in a 350-degree-F oven, covered, for 25 to 30 minutes, or until piping hot in center. (If desired, uncover and place briefly under broiler at the end of the cooking time.)

PER FILLED CREPE: CALORIES: 217; FAT: 7 G; CHOLESTEROL: 85 MG; SODIUM: 231 MG; PROTEIN: 19 G; CARBOHYDRATE: 19 G

# Meatballs with Parsley and Sage

*Cathy B.*

MAKES 28 MEATBALLS

**M**ADE WITH LEAN GROUND ROUND AND GRATED POTATOES, these meatballs are great plain, but they can also be dressed up with barbecue or sweet and sour sauce. (You may want to omit the sage if you plan to add the meatballs to spaghetti sauce with Italian herbs.) Ask your butcher to grind the round steak for you.

| | |
|---|---|
| 1½ | pounds round steak, trimmed of fat and ground |
| 1 | cup finely grated raw potatoes (about 8 ounces) |
| 2 | large eggs |
| 1 | small onion, finely chopped (about ⅓ cup) |
| ¼ | cup shredded Parmesan cheese (about 1 ounce) |
| 1 | tablespoon minced fresh parsley |
| 1 | tablespoon dried sage |
| 1 | large garlic clove, minced |
| 1 | teaspoon grated lemon rind |
| ½ | teaspoon salt |
| ⅛ | teaspoon ground nutmeg |
| | Generous grating black pepper |

1. Preheat oven to 350 degrees F. Spray a cookie sheet with nonstick cooking spray. Set aside.

2. Place all ingredients in a large bowl and thoroughly combine.

3. Shape into 1½-inch balls (about the size of golf balls). Place on prepared cookie sheet. Bake for 30 to 40 minutes, or until no trace of pink remains when a cut is made in center of meatball. Serve hot immediately, or add to a sauce and serve hot.

PER 2-MEATBALL SERVING: CALORIES: 90; FAT: 3 G; CHOLESTEROL: 59 MG; SODIUM: 133 MG; PROTEIN: 12 G; CARBOHYDRATE: 3 G

# Joy's Pepper Steak

*Joy C.*

SERVES 6

A SIMPLE CLASSIC, this pepper steak is great served on a bed of rice or noodles. Accompany with a cabbage salad, such as Confetti Cabbage Salad (page 271).

1    pound round steak, trimmed of fat
     and cut into bite-sized pieces
1    teaspoon garlic powder
     Generous grating black pepper
2    cans (15 ounces each) Italian stewed tomatoes
3    tablespoons tomato paste
1    cup defatted beef broth
1    tablespoon lemon juice
4    medium green bell peppers, cut into
     ¾-inch chunks (about 4 cups)
1    large onion, cut into 8 wedges
2    cans (4 ounces each) button mushrooms, drained

1. In a small bowl, toss round steak with garlic powder and pepper.

2. Spray a large nonstick skillet or Dutch oven with nonstick cooking spray. Add meat and brown over medium-high heat for 5 to 7 minutes, stirring frequently. Add tomatoes, tomato paste, broth and lemon juice. Bring to a boil, cover, reduce heat to low and simmer for 1 hour. Add green peppers, onion and mushrooms, cover and simmer for 20 minutes more, or until meat is tender. Serve immediately.

PER SERVING: CALORIES: 172; FAT: 3 G; CHOLESTEROL: 39 MG; SODIUM: 765 MG; PROTEIN: 19 G; CARBOHYDRATE: 20 G

# Lazy Beef Stroganoff

*Joy C.*

SERVES 6

THIS CREAMY, RICH-TASTING COMBINATION of stroganoff sauce, curly noodles and ground beef has just a fraction of the fat of the traditional version. It's a "fast-food" adaptation, because Ramen Noodles cook faster than egg noodles, which are usually used in stroganoff. Serve with a spinach salad and sliced beets.

¾    pound extra-lean ground beef
1    large onion, chopped (about 1 cup)
1    can (10¾ ounces) reduced-fat cream
     of mushroom soup
1    cup nonfat sour cream
1½   tablespoons Worcestershire sauce, or to taste
2    packages (3 ounces each) reduced-fat Ramen Noodles
     (discard seasoning packet), cooked according
     to package directions and drained
½    teaspoon paprika
¼    cup chopped fresh parsley
     Freshly ground black pepper

1. In a large nonstick skillet over medium-high heat, brown beef and onion for 7 to 9 minutes, or until no trace of pink remains in meat. Remove from heat; drain.

2. Over medium heat, stir in soup, sour cream and Worcestershire. Stir in noodles. Stirring frequently but gently, heat for 5 to 10 minutes, or until mixture is heated through and just beginning to bubble around edges. (If it seems too thick, add a little more beef broth or water.) Sprinkle with paprika, parsley and pepper and serve.

PER SERVING: CALORIES: 281; FAT: 6 G; CHOLESTEROL: 37 MG; SODIUM: 334 MG; PROTEIN: 19 G; CARBOHYDRATE: 36 G

# Easy Beef Stew

*Joy C.*

SERVES 6

THERE IS NO NEED to brown the meat for this simple oven stew, which makes a perfect one-pot meal. If you have any left, you can warm it as is or thin with some V-8 juice or broth and enjoy it as a soup. Joy notes that this stew is also good made with lean pork in place of the beef.

1   can (15 ounces) Italian stewed tomatoes
1⅓ cups water
½   cup beer
1½ pounds round steak, trimmed of all fat and
      cut into bite-sized pieces
1   medium onion, chopped (about ⅔ cup)
1   pound potatoes, cut into ½-inch cubes
      (about 4 medium)
3   cups frozen mixed vegetables (peas, corn,
      beans and carrots)
4   medium carrots, cut into bite-sized pieces
      (about 2 cups)
1   teaspoon dried basil
1   large garlic clove, minced
1   teaspoon salt
      Generous grating black pepper
2   tablespoons all-purpose flour

1. Preheat oven to 325 degrees F. In a large Dutch oven or casserole, combine tomatoes, 1 cup water, beer, meat and onion. Cover and bake for 1 hour, stirring occasionally.

2. Add remaining vegetables, basil, garlic, salt and pepper. Stir gently. Cover and bake for 1 hour more, or until meat is tender, stirring occasionally.

3. About ½ hour before stew is done, whisk remaining ⅓ cup water into flour in a small bowl. Stir flour mixture into stew. Return to oven, cover and bake for 20 to 30 minutes more, or until thickened, stirring several times. (Add more water if gravy is too thick.) Serve promptly.

PER SERVING: CALORIES: 312; FAT: 4 G; CHOLESTEROL: 59 MG; SODIUM: 632 MG;

PROTEIN: 30 G; CARBOHYDRATE: 40 G

# Sweet and Sour Pork

## JoAnna M. Lund

### SERVES 4

THIS SUPER-SIMPLE DISH is both lighter and more flavorful than the traditional Chinese version, which is made with deep-fried pork. JoAnna's recipe also eliminates the bother of making a sauce. The natural accompaniment for this dish is rice. (Chicken can be substituted for the pork.) This recipe was adapted from one in JoAnna Lund's *HELP: Healthy Exchanges Lifetime Plan* (G.P. Putnam's Sons).

¼ cup apple cider vinegar
1 can (15¼ ounces) juice-packed canned pineapple chunks, drained; juice reserved
1 tablespoon soy sauce
1 tablespoon cornstarch
¼ teaspoon ground ginger
 Generous grating black pepper
1 pound boneless pork sirloin, loin chops or pork tenderloin, trimmed of fat and cut into thin strips (about ½ x 2½ inches)
½ cup finely chopped onion
⅓ cup apricot preserves or spreadable fruit
1 large green and/or red bell pepper, cut into strips

1. In a small bowl, whisk together vinegar, ¼ cup pineapple juice, soy sauce, cornstarch, ginger and pepper. Set aside.

2. Spray a large nonstick skillet with nonstick cooking spray. Over medium-high heat, brown pork for 4 to 5 minutes.

3. Stir in onion and sauté for 1 to 2 minutes more, or until onion starts to become limp.

4. Whisk together pineapple-juice mixture and stir into pork-onion mixture. Add preserves or spreadable fruit and pepper strips, and bring to a boil, stirring constantly. Cook for 2 to 3 minutes more, or until pepper is just tender-crisp.

5. Gently mix in pineapple chunks, heat through and serve immediately.

PER SERVING: CALORIES: 338; FAT: 9 G; CHOLESTEROL: 71 MG; SODIUM: 331 MG;

PROTEIN: 25 G; CARBOHYDRATE: 41 G

# Grilled Honey-Dijon Pork

*Sam Eukel*

Serves 4 to 6

THIS FIT-FOR-COMPANY RECIPE is easy but fancy-tasting. I got rave reviews from guests when I served it along with fresh corn on the cob, Fruits and Greens in Raspberry Vinaigrette (page 283) and Green Bean-Almond Rice (page 297). This recipe was adapted from one in Sam Eukel's *Sensibly Thin: Low-Fat Living and Cooking, Volume II.*

2   tablespoons apricot jam (regular or all-fruit)
1   tablespoon Dijon-style mustard
1   tablespoon honey
1   tablespoon teriyaki or tamari sauce
3   large garlic cloves, minced
1¼  pounds whole pork tenderloin or boneless center-cut
    pork chops (⅝ to ¾ inch thick), trimmed of fat

1. In a small bowl, whisk together jam, mustard, honey, teriyaki or tamari sauce and garlic. Place in a shallow baking dish.

2. Add meat and turn to coat all sides. Cover and refrigerate for at least 2 hours or overnight, turning periodically. Reserve marinade.

3. Preheat a gas grill or prepare a charcoal fire.

4. Grill pork over a medium-high fire for 4 to 5 minutes on one side, then baste with reserved marinade and turn. Cook for 4 to 5 minutes more, then baste again. Turn and cook for 3 to 5 minutes more, until no trace of pink remains in middle or until an instant-read meat thermometer inserted into center registers 160 degrees F. Do not overcook. (Allow less time for thinner pork chops.) Serve immediately.

PER SERVING: CALORIES: 164; FAT: 5 G; CHOLESTEROL: 66 MG; SODIUM: 196 MG; PROTEIN: 22 G; CARBOHYDRATE: 8 G

# Cheddar Fish

*Paul A.*

SERVES 4

PAUL'S INSPIRATION for this recipe is a Newfoundland "cod au gratin" dish. His reasons for liking it are simple: "It's low in fat and calories, easy to make and tastes great!" He adds a British favorite to this dish: malt vinegar, which is made from malted barley and usually comes in a shaker bottle. It is found in the condiment section of some supermarkets.

1¼  pounds fresh or frozen (thawed) cod fillets,
   about ½ inch thick
2-3  tablespoons malt vinegar
½  cup shredded reduced-fat Cheddar cheese (2 ounces)

1. Spray a nonstick skillet with nonstick cooking spray and place on a hot burner. (If using an electric stove, preheat burner to medium-high.)

2. Add fish to pan and sprinkle liberally with malt vinegar. Cook for about 3 minutes, adding more vinegar as it evaporates in pan.

3. Turn fish over, and sprinkle with malt vinegar. Cook for about 2 minutes more, or until fish just starts to flake at thickest part. Sprinkle evenly with Cheddar cheese. Cover and cook until cheese is melted; don't overcook. Serve immediately.

PER SERVING: CALORIES: 157; FAT: 3 G; CHOLESTEROL: 69 MG; SODIUM: 161 MG;

PROTEIN: 29 G; CARBOHYDRATE: 1 G

# Pirate's Pie

*Sam Eukel*

SERVES 6

THIS RECIPE IS BASED ON a favorite of Sam's uncle, who, because
of his jolly, somewhat mischievous spirit and Navy background,
was nicknamed "the pirate." Weighing more than 300 pounds at
the end of his life, he wasn't into low-fat eating, so Sam "lightened up"
the original version of this tuna-crusted, mashed-potato-topped casserole "pie." This recipe was adapted from one in Sam Eukel's *Sensibly Thin: Low-Fat Living and Cooking, Volume II.*

|   |   |
|---|---|
| 2 | large egg whites |
| 1 | large egg |
| 1 | can (6 ounces) water-packed tuna, drained |
| 1 | can (7 ounces) sliced mushrooms, drained |
| ⅓ | cup unseasoned bread crumbs |
| ¼ | cup nonfat mayonnaise |
| 1 | tablespoon chopped green onion |
| 1 | tablespoon chopped fresh parsley |
|   | Generous grating black pepper |
| 1 | medium tomato (about 4 ounces), sliced |
| 4 | slices fat-free cheese |
| 3 | cups mashed potatoes (instant or homemade), made with skim milk and diet margarine |
| ¼ | cup shredded reduced-fat Cheddar cheese (about 1 ounce) |

1. Preheat oven to 375 degrees F. Spray a 9-inch pie pan with nonstick
cooking spray; set aside.

2. In a medium bowl, with a fork, slightly beat egg whites and egg
together. Mix in tuna, mushrooms, bread crumbs, mayonnaise, green
onion, parsley and pepper until well combined. Pat into pie pan.

3. Top tuna mixture evenly with tomato slices, then cheese slices. Spoon mashed potatoes evenly over top and seal edges to prevent filling from leaking out. Sprinkle with Cheddar cheese.

4. Bake for 25 to 30 minutes, or until potatoes become golden brown around edges and casserole is piping hot in center. Serve immediately.

PER SERVING: CALORIES: 226; FAT: 7 G; CHOLESTEROL: 15 MG; SODIUM: 852 MG; PROTEIN: 15 G; CARBOHYDRATE: 26 G

# Shrimp and Pepper Mexicana

*Keith Van Gasken*

SERVES 4

LIME JUICE, CUMIN, CILANTRO AND GARLIC nicely complement the shrimp. Serve this festive-looking dish over rice or pasta, and if desired, top with a little salsa.

2   large tomatoes, chopped (about 2 cups)
⅓   cup chopped fresh cilantro
1   large garlic clove, minced
1   teaspoon ground cumin
½   teaspoon salt
¼   teaspoon cayenne pepper
    Juice of 1 lime (about ¼ cup)
1   pound medium shrimp, shelled and deveined
½   cup defatted chicken broth
1   large red bell pepper, cut into strips
1   large green bell pepper, cut into strips
1   large yellow bell pepper, cut into strips
1   medium onion, peeled and sliced lengthwise
½   cup sliced black olives (2 ounces)

1. In a medium nonaluminum bowl, stir together tomatoes, cilantro, garlic, cumin, salt, cayenne pepper and lime juice. Set aside.

2. Steam shrimp by placing them in a large covered pot with a shallow amount of boiling water. After water returns to a boil, steam shrimp until pink, 2 to 3 minutes. Drain. While they are still hot, toss gently with tomato mixture. Cover with plastic wrap and marinate in refrigerator for 15 minutes to 1 hour.

3. In a large nonstick skillet, bring broth to a boil, add peppers and onion and stir-fry over medium-high heat until tender-crisp, 5 to 7 minutes. Add shrimp mixture to peppers and heat through for 2 to 3 minutes, being careful not to overcook shrimp. Sprinkle with olives and serve immediately.

PER SERVING: CALORIES: 166; FAT: 3 G; CHOLESTEROL: 137 MG; SODIUM: 658 MG; PROTEIN: 18 G; CARBOHYDRATE: 19 G

# Spicy Shrimp and Cauliflower

*Lolly D.*

SERVES 6

THIS FLAVORFUL COMBINATION of shrimp, tomatoes and cauliflower is especially good served over linguine. (For added color, try spinach linguine.) Top with a little Parmesan cheese, and serve with a green salad and toasted rolls—cut in half, lightly sprayed with olive oil spray and sprinkled with garlic salt.

| | |
|---|---|
| 1¼ | pounds medium shrimp, shelled and deveined |
| 1 | tablespoon olive oil |
| 1 | large onion, chopped (about 1 cup) |
| 1 | large garlic clove, minced |
| 1 | large carrot, sliced into ⅛-inch coins (about 1 cup) |
| 1 | can (28 ounces) stewed tomatoes |
| 1 | bottle (8 ounces) clam juice |
| ½ | cup defatted chicken broth |
| ¼ | teaspoon ground cumin |
| ¼ | teaspoon red pepper flakes |
| ¼ | teaspoon dried thyme |
| 1 | tablespoon lemon juice |
| 5 | tablespoons tomato paste |
| | Generous grating black pepper |
| 1 | small cauliflower (about 1 pound), cut into bite-sized pieces |

1. Steam shrimp by placing them in a large covered pot with a small amount of boiling water. After water returns to a boil, steam shrimp until pink, 2 to 3 minutes. Drain and run cold water over shrimp so they don't cook further.

2. Heat oil in a large nonstick skillet over medium-high heat. Sauté onion and garlic for 2 to 3 minutes, until limp. (Don't brown.) Add carrot, tomatoes, clam juice, broth, cumin, red pepper, thyme, lemon juice, tomato paste and pepper. Cover and simmer for about 12 minutes.

3. Add cauliflower, cover and cook for 5 minutes, or until cauliflower is tender-crisp. Stir in shrimp until just heated through. Serve immediately.

PER SERVING: CALORIES: 231; FAT 7 G; CHOLESTEROL: 115 MG; SODIUM: 1,012 MG; PROTEIN: 18 G; CARBOHYDRATE: 27 G

# Linguine with Fresh Tomatoes

*Don Mauer*

SERVES 6

COOKED LINGUINE marinates in a garlicky, fresh tomato-basil sauce with a splash of red wine vinegar and a touch of olive oil. If you like, you can also dust this dish with a touch of freshly grated Parmesan.

2 tablespoons olive oil (preferably extra-virgin)
6 large garlic cloves, minced
3 pounds very ripe tomatoes, coarsely chopped, liquid reserved (about 6 cups)
½ cup chopped fresh basil leaves or 1 tablespoon dried plus 1 teaspoon
3 tablespoons red wine vinegar or 1 tablespoon balsamic vinegar
1 teaspoon salt
½ teaspoon freshly ground black pepper
1 pound dried linguine

1. Heat 1 tablespoon oil in a small nonstick skillet over medium heat. Add garlic and cook, stirring, for 2 to 3 minutes; do not brown. Transfer garlic and oil to a large nonaluminum bowl.

2. Add tomatoes and reserved liquid, basil, vinegar, remaining 1 tablespoon oil, salt and pepper, stirring to combine. Cover and let stand at room temperature for 1 to 2 hours so flavors blend.

3. Just before serving, cook linguine according to package directions, until hard center is gone but pasta is still chewy, about 10 minutes. Drain well. Transfer to large bowl with sauce. Toss until sauce is evenly distributed throughout linguine.

PER SERVING: CALORIES: 389; FAT: 7 G; CHOLESTEROL: 0 MG; SODIUM: 587 MG; PROTEIN: 12 G; CARBOHYDRATE: 71 G

# Zesty Pasta Sauce

*Randy W.*

SERVES 4; MAKES ABOUT 3 CUPS

ANDY PREFERS TO USE FRESH HERBS in this spicy pasta sauce, which is embellished with black olives and Parmesan cheese. Red pepper flakes give it a zing. Serve over your favorite pasta or with chicken or fish.

1 tablespoon olive oil
1 medium onion, chopped (⅔ cup)
4 large garlic cloves, minced
1 can (28 ounces) diced tomatoes, with juice
1 tablespoon minced fresh marjoram or 1 teaspoon dried
1 tablespoon minced fresh thyme or 1 teaspoon dried
1 tablespoon minced fresh oregano or 1 teaspoon dried
2 tablespoons minced fresh basil or 2 teaspoons dried
1 bay leaf
¼ teaspoon red pepper flakes
¼ teaspoon white pepper
¼ cup shredded Parmesan cheese (about 1 ounce)
½ cup sliced black olives (about 2 ounces)

1. In a large nonstick skillet or Dutch oven, heat oil over medium-high heat. Add onion and garlic and sauté until onion is transparent but not brown. Add tomatoes and juice, reduce heat to low and simmer uncovered for 20 minutes.

2. Stir in herbs, red pepper flakes and white pepper. Simmer, partially covered, for another 20 minutes. (At this point, you can refrigerate sauce until ready to serve.) Just before serving, remove bay leaf. Reheat if necessary, then stir in Parmesan and olives. Serve hot.

PER SERVING: CALORIES: 137; FAT: 7 G; CHOLESTEROL: 4 MG; SODIUM: 639 MG;

PROTEIN: 4 G; CARBOHYDRATE: 18 G

# Garden Vegetable Sauce for Pasta

*Stephanie C.*

MAKES APPROXIMATELY 10 SERVINGS, EACH 1 CUP

THIS CHUNKY SAUCE makes a large quantity and freezes well—keep it on hand for impromptu entertaining. Stephanie suggests topping your favorite pasta with a dollop of low-fat ricotta cheese, then adding her sauce. This recipe, which has been slightly adapted, received honorable mention in a 1992 cookoff sponsored by the *Daily Freeman* of Kingston, New York.

1 tablespoon olive oil
1 large onion, chopped (1 cup)
4 large garlic cloves, minced
2 medium zucchini (14-16 ounces total),
   cut into ¼-inch slices
1 large eggplant (16 ounces), peeled and
   cut into ½-inch cubes
2 cans (28 ounces each) crushed tomatoes
1 can (15 ounces) tomato sauce
1 can (6 ounces) tomato paste
½ cup Burgundy
⅓ cup water
2 tablespoons granulated sugar
1 tablespoon chopped fresh parsley or
   1 teaspoon dried flakes
1 teaspoon dried basil

1. In a 6-quart nonaluminum pot, heat oil over medium-high heat. Add onion and sauté, stirring frequently, for 4 to 5 minutes, or until onion is limp but not brown. Add garlic and sauté for about 1 minute more, until softened.

2. Add all remaining ingredients and blend well. Bring to a boil, stirring frequently. Reduce heat to low and simmer, partially covered, for 2 hours, stirring occasionally. Serve immediately or cool, then freeze in airtight containers.

PER SERVING: CALORIES: 121; FAT: 2 G; CHOLESTEROL: 0 MG; SODIUM: 740 MG;

PROTEIN: 4 G; CARBOHYDRATE: 24 G

# Shells Stuffed with Ricotta and Zucchini

*Ann F.*

SERVES 6

KIDS AND ADULTS ALIKE love these pasta shells, which are filled with a ricotta-cheese mixture speckled with zucchini and topped with low-fat spaghetti sauce, allowing you to "sneak" in a green vegetable for finicky eaters. Serve with warm Italian bread and Perfect Caesar Salad (page 272).

18-20   dried jumbo pasta shells (about 7 ounces)
   1   large shallot, chopped
   1   container (15 ounces) nonfat ricotta cheese
   1   large zucchini (about 9 ounces), shredded
      and squeezed gently to drain juice
   1   container (4 ounces) refrigerated or frozen egg
      substitute (thawed) or 2 large eggs, lightly beaten
  ¼   teaspoon ground nutmeg
   1   jar (26 ounces) reduced-fat spaghetti sauce
  ¼   cup shredded Parmesan cheese (1 ounce)

1. Spray a casserole dish (11 x 7 inches or 9 x 13 inches) with nonstick cooking spray. Set aside. Preheat oven to 350 degrees F.

2. Cook pasta shells according to package directions, until tender, about 12 minutes, then drain and set aside.

3. Meanwhile, spray a small skillet with nonstick cooking spray. Add shallot and sauté over medium heat until limp but not brown. Remove from heat. In a medium bowl, with a fork, stir together shallot, ricotta, zucchini, egg substitute or eggs and nutmeg until well blended. Set aside.

4. Spread 2 cups spaghetti sauce over bottom of casserole dish. With a spoon, fill each shell with about 2 tablespoons ricotta filling. Set shells in casserole dish.

5. Top with remaining spaghetti sauce. Bake, covered, for 30 minutes. Uncover, sprinkle with Parmesan, and bake for 10 to 15 minutes more, or until shells are piping hot in middle. Serve promptly.

PER SERVING: CALORIES: 277; FAT: 3 G; CHOLESTEROL: 7 MG; SODIUM: 486 MG; PROTEIN: 20 G; CARBOHYDRATE: 39 G

# Chicken and Peppers with Penne Pasta

*Michael F.*

SERVES 4

I LOVE THE APPEARANCE—and the taste—of this simple-to-make dish: penne pasta topped with tomatoes, then with sautéed chicken strips and red and green peppers. Serve with warm Italian bread and a tossed salad. If desired, sprinkle each serving with Parmesan or Romano cheese.

12 ounces boneless, skinless chicken breasts,
   cut into ½-x-2-inch strips
1 cup defatted chicken broth
8 ounces dried penne pasta
1 medium green bell pepper
1 medium red bell pepper
1 can (14½ ounces) Italian-seasoned tomatoes,
   cut into bite-sized chunks, juice reserved
1 tablespoon diet margarine
1 large garlic clove, minced
1 tablespoon chopped fresh parsley or
   1 teaspoon dried flakes
½ teaspoon salt
¼ teaspoon freshly ground black pepper

1. Marinate chicken in broth in refrigerator for at least 1 hour.

2. Cook pasta according to package directions, until hard center is gone but pasta is still chewy, about 10 minutes. Drain and set aside.

3. Cut peppers into 1-inch diamond shapes or squares. Set aside.

4. In a small saucepan, bring tomatoes to a boil over medium-high heat. Turn heat to low and cover saucepan, leaving tomatoes on burner until ready to serve.

5. Melt margarine in skillet over medium-high heat. Turn heat to high and add chicken (discard marinade broth). Quick-fry until chicken pieces are lightly browned, 3 to 4 minutes. Reduce heat to medium-high and add reserved peppers, garlic, parsley, salt and pepper. Cook, stirring frequently, for about 5 minutes more, or until no trace of pink remains when you cut into thickest part of chicken.

6. Divide pasta into 4 equal portions in large, shallow bowls. Spoon one-fourth of hot tomatoes over each pasta serving and top with one-fourth of chicken-and-pepper mixture. Serve immediately.

Per serving: calories: 388; fat: 5 g; cholesterol: 58 mg; sodium: 590 mg; protein: 25 g; carbohydrate: 55 g

# Party Turkey Tetrazzini

*JoAnna M. Lund*

SERVES 4

$\mathbb{S}$ PAGHETTI, LOW-FAT CHEDDAR CHEESE, turkey breast and reduced-fat cream of mushroom soup are blended in this creamy
low-fat version of the traditional rendition, which is made with
heavy cream and several tablespoons of butter. In JoAnna's version,
chopped pimiento and parsley add an attractive confetti-like touch.
Serve with a fresh fruit salad and warm low-fat biscuits. This recipe
was adapted from one in JoAnna Lund's *Healthy Exchanges Cookbook*
(G.P. Putnam's Sons).

4    ounces dried spaghetti, broken into thirds
½    cup chopped onion
1    can (10¾ ounces) Campbell's Healthy Request
     Cream of Mushroom Soup
½    cup skim milk
¾    cup shredded reduced-fat Cheddar cheese (3 ounces)
8    ounces cooked skinless turkey breast,
     cut into ½-x-2-inch strips (about 1½ cups)
2    tablespoons chopped pimiento
2    tablespoons chopped fresh parsley or
     2 teaspoons dried flakes
     Generous grating black pepper

1. In a large pot of boiling water, cook spaghetti according to package directions until tender but still firm, about 10 minutes. Drain and
set aside.

2. Spray a large nonstick skillet with nonstick cooking spray. Add onion
and sauté over medium-high heat until tender, about 3 minutes.

3. Reduce heat to medium. Stir in soup, milk and Cheddar cheese. Cook, stirring frequently, until cheese is melted, 5 to 8 minutes.

4. Gently mix in spaghetti, turkey, pimiento, parsley and pepper. Cook, stirring often, until mixture is heated through, 3 to 5 minutes. Serve promptly in shallow bowls.

**Make-ahead oven method:** Follow steps 1 and 2, then place mixture in a 2-quart casserole dish sprayed with nonstick cooking spray. Cover and refrigerate. Preheat oven to 350 degrees F and bake covered casserole for 15 minutes. Uncover and bake for 20 to 30 minutes more, or until casserole is heated through and mixture starts to bubble. Serve hot.

PER SERVING: CALORIES: 296; FAT: 6 G; CHOLESTEROL: 63 MG; SODIUM: 553 MG; PROTEIN: 28 G; CARBOHYDRATE: 30 G

# Vegetable Lasagna

*Keith Van Gasken*

SERVES 10

KEITH'S LOADED-WITH-VEGETABLES meatless lasagna is filling
and appealing to vegetarians and carnivores alike. To save time
(and clean-up), the lasagna noodles are not precooked; they cook
in the vegetable juices. The recipe makes a large quantity, so it's great
for a crowd or if you want leftovers.

¼  cup dry white wine or water
2  boxes (10 ounces each) frozen chopped spinach,
    thawed, or defrosted in microwave and drained
1  pound mushrooms, cleaned and sliced (5-6 cups)
1  extra-large onion, chopped (about 1½ cups)
1  large green bell pepper, chopped (about 1½ cups)
1  container (24 ounces) nonfat cottage cheese
4  large egg whites
1  teaspoon garlic powder
1  teaspoon dried basil
1  teaspoon dried oregano
1  jar (26 ounces) plus 1 cup reduced-fat spaghetti sauce
8  ounces dried lasagna noodles
1  cup shredded part-skim mozzarella cheese (4 ounces)

1. Preheat oven to 375 degrees F. Spray a 9-x-13-inch pan with nonstick cooking spray. Set aside. Heat wine or water in a large skillet or
pot over medium-high heat. Add spinach, mushrooms, onion and
green pepper and sauté for 7 to 10 minutes, or until vegetables just begin to become limp. Remove from heat and drain thoroughly. Set
aside.

2. In a large bowl, mixing by hand, combine cottage cheese, egg
whites, garlic powder, basil and oregano. Add reserved vegetable mixture and mix gently. Set aside.

3. Spread 1⅓ cups spaghetti sauce evenly over bottom of pan. Top with one-third of uncooked noodles, then spread with one-third of vegetable-cheese mixture. Repeat one more time. For final layer, add remaining noodles, then spread with remaining vegetable mixture. Top with remaining spaghetti sauce. Sprinkle with mozzarella.

4. Cover with foil and bake for 45 minutes. (Try not to let the cover touch cheese.) Uncover and bake for 15 to 20 minutes more, or until piping hot in center. Let stand for 15 minutes before serving, so lasagna sets. (To store, allow pan of lasagna to cool, then cover tightly with plastic wrap and refrigerate or freeze.)

PER SERVING: CALORIES: 260; FAT: 3 G; CHOLESTEROL: 11 MG; SODIUM: 435 MG; PROTEIN: 22 G; CARBOHYDRATE: 35 G

# Best Macaroni and Cheese

*Diane J.*

SERVES 8

PUREED COTTAGE CHEESE makes a smooth sauce base for a mixture of macaroni, reduced-fat Cheddar cheese and onion. Diane adds distinctive flavors with bacon bits, Dijon mustard and fresh parsley. I've never tasted a better reduced-fat macaroni and cheese. Serve as a side dish or a main meal.

This dish can be made ahead, covered and refrigerated. When ready to cook, preheat oven to 350 degrees F. Cook, covered, for 20 minutes. Uncover and cook for 15 minutes more, or until piping hot in the center.

| | |
|---|---|
| 7 | ounces (about 1¾ cups) dried macaroni |
| 2 | cups shredded reduced-fat sharp Cheddar cheese (8 ounces) |
| ½ | cup finely chopped onion |
| 3 | tablespoons chopped fresh parsley |
| ½ | teaspoon freshly ground black pepper |
| 1¾ | cups nonfat cottage cheese |
| ½ | cup evaporated skim milk |
| 2 | teaspoons Dijon-style mustard |
| 2 | tablespoons bacon bits |
| ⅓ | cup unseasoned bread crumbs |
| 3 | tablespoons shredded Parmesan cheese |

1. In a large pot of boiling water, cook macaroni according to package directions, until tender but firm, about 8 minutes. Drain.

2. Preheat oven to 350 degrees F. Spray a 2-quart casserole with nonstick cooking spray; set aside. In a large bowl, gently combine cooked macaroni, Cheddar cheese, onion, parsley and pepper.

3. In a blender or a food processor, combine cottage cheese, milk and mustard. Process until smooth. Pour over macaroni mixture and mix thoroughly. Turn into prepared casserole.

4. In a small bowl, blend bacon bits, bread crumbs and Parmesan. Sprinkle over top of macaroni. Bake, uncovered, for 20 to 25 minutes, or until hot in center. Serve hot.

PER SERVING: CALORIES: 248; FAT: 7 G; CHOLESTEROL: 20 MG; SODIUM: 308 MG; PROTEIN: 17 G; CARBOHYDRATE: 27 G

# Ham, Swiss and Spinach Calzones

*Diane J.*

MAKES 6 CALZONES

TRADITIONAL CALZONES, which are stuffed pizzas that look like turnovers, are filled with fatty cheeses. Diane saves many fat grams by making this filling with spinach, lean ham and reduced-fat cheese. (My kids, who won't touch plain spinach, loved this recipe.) The calzones can also be filled with Mushroom-Sausage Filling (page 252). Serve with fresh grapes, carrot sticks and a glass of skim milk.

FILLING

5   ounces (½ a 10-ounce package) frozen chopped spinach, cooked according to package directions and squeezed of excess moisture
¾   cup finely chopped extra-lean cooked ham (about 4 ounces)
¾   cup shredded reduced-fat Swiss cheese (3 ounces)
2   tablespoons thinly sliced green onion

CRUST

1   package (10 ounces) refrigerated pizza dough, such as Pillsbury All Ready Pizza Crust
1   large egg
2   tablespoons shredded Parmesan cheese

1. **To make filling**: In a medium bowl, combine spinach, ham, cheese and green onion. Set aside.

2. Preheat oven to 425 degrees F. Spray a baking sheet with nonstick cooking spray. Set aside.

3. **To make crust**: Unroll pizza dough on a lightly floured work surface. Roll or stretch dough into a 15-x-10-inch rectangle. Cut into six 5-inch squares.

4. Place ⅓ cup filling in center of each square. Brush all 4 edges with water. Bring one corner of dough up and over filling, pressing into dough on other side of filling. Repeat with opposite side of dough, pressing with a fork or finger to seal as you go. Continue with remaining two corners. (Calzones will be square.) Make sure there are no holes or cracks.

5. Arrange seam side down on prepared baking sheet. Prick tops with a fork. Set aside.

6. In a small bowl, whisk together egg and 1 teaspoon water; brush onto tops of calzones. Sprinkle with Parmesan. Bake for 8 to 10 minutes, or until golden brown. Calzones are best served immediately, but they can be cooled, wrapped tightly and reheated in the oven or a microwave.

PER CALZONE: CALORIES: 207; FAT: 5 G; CHOLESTEROL: 35 MG; SODIUM: 654 MG;

PROTEIN: 13 G; CARBOHYDRATE: 26 G

# Mushroom-Sausage Filling for Calzones

*Diane J.*

MAKES ENOUGH FILLING FOR 6 CALZONES

T HIS FILLING FOR CALZONES tastes like a traditional cheese-and-sausage pizza topping but is lower in fat, because lean pork chops are used in place of sausage. To prepare calzones and bake, see pages 250 and 251.

8    ounces boneless extra-lean pork chops,
      trimmed and ground
4    ounces fresh mushrooms, sliced (about 1 cup)
¾    cup reduced-fat pizza sauce
½    teaspoon garlic powder
½    teaspoon fennel seeds
      Freshly ground black pepper
¾    cup shredded part-skim mozzarella cheese (3 ounces)

1. Spray a large nonstick skillet with nonstick cooking spray. Over medium-high heat, cook pork, stirring, for 5 to 7 minutes, or until no trace of pink remains. Add mushrooms and cook until slightly wilted, 2 to 3 minutes. Stir in pizza sauce, garlic powder, fennel seeds and pepper. Bring to a boil, stirring frequently, then lower heat and simmer, uncovered, for 5 minutes.

2. Remove from heat and stir in mozzarella until melted. Divide filling evenly among calzones.

PER CALZONE: CALORIES: 258; FAT: 8 G; CHOLESTEROL: 50 MG; SODIUM: 543 MG; PROTEIN: 18 G; CARBOHYDRATE: 28 G

# Denver Pizza

*JoAnna M. Lund*

**A**FTER TRYING THIS COLORFUL PIZZA, you may never want the "real thing" again. This was adapted from a recipe in JoAnna Lund's *Healthy Exchanges Cookbook* (G.P. Putnam's Sons).

| | |
|---|---|
| 1 | can (11 ounces) refrigerated French bread dough |
| 2 | tablespoons mustard, preferably Dijon-style |
| 12 | ounces extra-lean cooked ham, finely diced (2 heaping cups) |
| 1¼ | cups chopped fresh mushrooms (about 4 ounces) |
| 1 | medium green bell pepper, chopped (about 1 cup) |
| 1 | cup diced fresh tomato |
| ½ | cup chopped onion |
| 1½ | cups shredded part-skim mozzarella cheese (6 ounces) |
| 1 | tablespoon chopped fresh parsley or 1 teaspoon dried |

1. Preheat oven to 375 degrees F. Spray a jellyroll pan with nonstick cooking spray. Unroll bread dough and pat into pan and up sides to form a rim.

2. Spread mustard evenly over crust. Sprinkle with a layer of ham, mushrooms, green pepper, tomato and onion. Sprinkle mozzarella and parsley evenly over top.

3. Bake for 15 to 20 minutes, or until cheese is bubbly. (Drain any excess moisture on top of pizza immediately.) Cool for 4 to 5 minutes before cutting into 8 pieces.

PER PIECE: CALORIES: 238; FAT: 7 G; CHOLESTEROL: 32 MG; SODIUM: 997 MG; PROTEIN: 18 G; CARBOHYDRATE: 25 G

# Cheesy Chili Mac

*Mary Ann K.*

MAKES 6 TO 8 SERVINGS

THIS MACARONI AND CHEESE WITH CHILI makes an easy last-minute main dish. Serve with a spinach salad and some crusty bread. (The dish can be made ahead of time by layering macaroni, sauce and cheese in a casserole dish, then heating in the oven just before serving.)

| | |
|---|---|
| 1 | pound ground uncooked turkey breast |
| 1 | envelope chili seasoning mix (check labels for lower-sodium brands) |
| 1 | can (14½ ounces) diced tomatoes |
| 1 | small can (8 ounces) tomato sauce |
| ½ | cup water |
| 1 | package (8 ounces) dried macaroni |
| 1½ | cups shredded reduced-fat Cheddar cheese (6 ounces) |

1. Coat a large nonstick skillet with nonstick cooking spray. Brown turkey over medium-high heat, mashing with fork to break up lumps.

2. Add chili seasoning mix, tomatoes, tomato sauce and water. Reduce heat to medium-low and simmer, uncovered, for about 20 minutes.

3. Meanwhile, in a large pot of boiling water, cook macaroni according to package directions—but omitting salt—until tender but firm, about 8 minutes. Drain.

4. Divide hot macaroni among 6 to 8 plates, depending on desired serving size. Spoon turkey mixture over macaroni and top each serving with Cheddar cheese. Serve immediately.

PER SERVING: CALORIES: 280; FAT: 5 G; CHOLESTEROL: 59 MG; SODIUM: 878 MG; PROTEIN: 26 G; CARBOHYDRATE: 30 G

# Easy Three-Bean Chili

*Barbara M.*

SERVES 6

THIS STRICTLY VEGETARIAN CHILI is a crowd pleaser and easy to make. It's even better served the next day, after the spices have had time to meld. If desired, top with shredded nonfat cheese and a dollop of nonfat sour cream.

1   medium green bell pepper, chopped (about 1 cup)
1   medium onion, chopped (about ⅔ cup)
2   medium garlic cloves, minced
1   can (15½ ounces) red kidney beans, drained
1   can (15½ ounces) great northern beans, drained
1   can (15½ ounces) chick-peas, drained
1   can (14½ ounces) stewed tomatoes,
      Cajun- or Mexican-style
2   cans (8 ounces each) tomato sauce
1   tablespoon chili powder
1   teaspoon granulated sugar
1   teaspoon dried basil
1   cup water
1-2   tablespoons apple cider vinegar (optional)

1. Coat a large nonstick Dutch oven or nonstick pot with nonstick cooking spray. Add green pepper, onion and garlic and sauté over medium-high heat for about 5 minutes, or until vegetables are soft but not brown.

2. Add beans, chick-peas, tomatoes, tomato sauce, chili powder, sugar, basil, water and vinegar, if using. Cover and simmer for 15 minutes, stirring occasionally. Serve hot in soup bowls.

PER SERVING: CALORIES: 284; FAT: 2 G; CHOLESTEROL: 0 MG; SODIUM: 1,223 MG; PROTEIN: 15 G; CARBOHYDRATE: 55 G

# Vegetarian Mexican "Lasagna"

*Diane J.*

SERVES 8 GENEROUSLY

A TASTY WAY TO BOOST YOUR INTAKE OF LEGUMES, this Mexican "lasagna" could easily be a meal in itself. Corn tortillas are layered with cheese and a tomato-mushroom-bean mixture—all seasoned with chili powder and cumin. Top each serving with shredded lettuce and a spoonful of salsa or picante sauce. It's nicely complemented by fresh fruit cocktail.

1   medium onion, chopped (⅔ cup)
2   cans (14½ ounces each) diced tomatoes, with juice
1   can (4 ounces) diced mild green chilies, drained
8   ounces fresh mushrooms, cleaned and sliced
1   can (15 ounces) kidney beans, drained
1   can (15 ounces) pinto beans, drained
1   can (6 ounces) tomato paste
1   tablespoon chili powder
1   teaspoon ground cumin
12  (5½-inch) corn tortillas (10-ounce package),
    cut in half
2   cups shredded reduced-fat Cheddar cheese
    (8 ounces)
1   cup nonfat sour cream

1. Preheat oven to 350 degrees F. Coat a 9-x-13-inch pan with nonstick cooking spray. Set aside.

2. Spray a large nonstick skillet with nonstick cooking spray. Add onion and sauté over medium-high heat until soft but not browned, 3 to 4 minutes.

3. Add tomatoes, chilies, mushrooms, beans, tomato paste, chili powder and cumin. Bring to a boil, stirring frequently, then reduce heat and simmer, uncovered, for 10 minutes.

4. Arrange 4 tortillas in prepared pan, cutting them to fit, if necessary, and overlapping them slightly. Spread one-third of tomato-bean mixture over tortillas. Sprinkle with one-third of Cheddar cheese. Repeat one more time. For third and final layer, arrange remaining tortillas, then spread with sour cream and top with remaining tomato-bean mixture. Sprinkle with remaining cheese. Bake for 30 minutes, or until cheese begins to brown and liquid is bubbling. Let rest for 15 minutes, then cut into 8 pieces and serve.

PER SERVING: CALORIES: 337; FAT: 7 G; CHOLESTEROL: 20 MG; SODIUM: 1,326 MG; PROTEIN: 24 G; CARBOHYDRATE: 49 G

# King Oskar's Chili

*Ken H.*

SERVES 6

THIS HEARTY, CHUNKY CHILI, made with stewed tomatoes and tomato soup, is part of the legacy of Ken H., who passed away since contacting me as a master. If you like a sweeter chili, add a tablespoon of brown sugar or one packet of low-calorie sweetener.

1 pound extra-lean ground beef
2 large celery stalks, chopped (about 1½ cups)
1 large green bell pepper, chopped (about 1½ cups)
1 medium onion, chopped (about ⅔ cup)
1 can (14½ ounces) stewed tomatoes, with juice
1 can (15½ ounces) kidney beans, with juice
1 can (10¾ ounces) tomato soup
2 tablespoons chili powder
⅛ teaspoon ground cloves
  Generous grating black pepper
  Hot sauce, to taste

1. Coat a large nonstick pot with nonstick cooking spray. Brown ground beef over medium-high heat, stirring frequently and breaking up chunks, for 8 to 10 minutes, or until no trace of pink remains. Drain off any fat.

2. Reduce heat to medium. Add celery, green pepper and onion. Cover and cook for 5 to 7 minutes, stirring occasionally, until vegetables are tender.

3. Add tomatoes, beans, tomato soup, chili powder, cloves and pepper. Lower heat, cover and simmer for 30 to 45 minutes, stirring occasionally. Add hot sauce and adjust seasonings to taste. Serve hot in soup bowls.

PER SERVING: CALORIES: 225; FAT: 6 G; CHOLESTEROL: 35 MG; SODIUM: 852 MG;

PROTEIN: 18 G; CARBOHYDRATE: 28 G

# Soft-Shell Turkey Tacos

*Diane J.*

SERVES 4

H ERE'S A DINNER that can be made ahead: a tasty combination of broccoli, cheese, ground turkey and Mexican flavorings, all rolled up in a warm tortilla. Serve with sliced pears and orange sections on a bed of lettuce. (If you like, just before serving, the tortillas can be topped with a spoonful of nonfat sour cream.)

| | |
|---|---|
| 4 | large (9-to-10 inch) flour tortillas |
| ¼ | cup nonfat salad dressing (Diane likes Miracle Whip Free) |
| ¼ | pound ground uncooked turkey breast |
| 2 | medium garlic cloves, minced |
| 6 | tablespoons salsa |
| | Generous grating black pepper |
| ½-1 | teaspoon chili powder |
| 1 | tablespoon chopped jalapeño pepper (fresh or from a jar or can) |
| 2 | cups broccoli florets, steamed |
| 1 | cup shredded reduced-fat Monterey Jack cheese (4 ounces) |

1. Spread each tortilla with 1 tablespoon dressing; set aside.

2. Spray a medium skillet with nonstick cooking spray. Brown turkey over medium heat for about 5 minutes, or until no trace of pink remains. Stir in garlic, 2 tablespoons salsa, pepper, chili powder to taste, jalapeño pepper and broccoli. Cook for 1 to 2 minutes, or just to heat through.

3. Preheat oven to 350 degrees F.

4. Distribute about one-fourth of turkey-broccoli mixture and cheese evenly over each tortilla. Top each tortilla with 1 tablespoon salsa and roll up to enclose filling. Place in a baking dish, cover tightly and warm for about 10 minutes in oven. Or reheat briefly for 15 to 20 seconds on high power in the microwave. (*These can be made ahead and refrigerated immediately after they are rolled, then warmed later in a preheated oven for about 20 minutes or in a microwave for 3 minutes, or until heated through.*) Serve immediately.

PER SERVING: CALORIES: 301; FAT: 9 G; CHOLESTEROL: 39 MG; SODIUM: 541 MG; PROTEIN: 22 G; CARBOHYDRATE: 34 G

# Vegetable Tofu Stir-Fry

*Dorothy C.*

SERVES 6 AS A MAIN DISH

DOROTHY IS RIGHT when she says this dish is "an extremely healthful and satisfying meal." The colorful mix of broccoli, carrots, peppers, mushrooms and bean sprouts is rounded out with tofu cubes and hearty brown rice—all seasoned with lemon pepper, white wine and soy sauce. She usually makes a double batch and saves some for leftovers the next day. (Frozen vegetables may be substituted for fresh, but they need to be drained after stir-frying to reduce sogginess.)

1   cup uncooked long-grain brown or white rice
1   tablespoon vegetable oil
2   cups broccoli florets
1   heaping cup sliced fresh mushrooms (about 4 ounces)
1   cup thinly sliced carrots (about 3 medium)
1   cup mung bean sprouts
1   medium red or green bell pepper, sliced into thin strips
½   cup chopped onion
¼   cup white wine
1   package (10 ounces) firm tofu, cut into ½-inch cubes
1   teaspoon lemon pepper
3   tablespoons tamari or soy sauce

1. To cook rice: Bring 2½ cups water (2 cups, if using white rice) to a boil. Add rice, stir once, then reduce heat to low. Cover and simmer for 45 to 50 minutes (18 to 20 minutes for white rice), or until rice is tender but firm and water has been absorbed. (You need about 3 cups cooked rice; you may have a little left over.) Remove from heat and set aside.

2. In a large nonstick skillet or a wok, heat oil over high heat. (Watch closely to avoid burning.) Add all vegetables and stir-fry for 2 minutes. (Lower heat if vegetables start to stick.) Sprinkle with wine. Stir-fry vegetables for about 3 minutes more, or until they start to become tender-crisp.

3. Reduce heat to medium, and gently stir in rice, tofu, lemon pepper and tamari or soy sauce. Stir until heated through, 3 to 5 minutes. Serve immediately.

PER SERVING: CALORIES: 233; FAT: 7 G; CHOLESTEROL: 0 MG; SODIUM: 618 MG;

PROTEIN: 12 G; CARBOHYDRATE: 31 G

# Vegetarian Chow Mein

*Arlene Z.*

THIS MEATLESS CHINESE-TYPE DISH is laden with chopped celery, onion, green and red bell peppers, mushrooms, snow peas and water chestnuts in a garlicky soy-cornstarch sauce. Since the recipe is virtually fat-free, you can spend a few grams of fat on a light topping of crisp chow mein noodles. Serve over rice.

2 cups vegetable (or chicken) broth
¼ cup cornstarch
3 cups chopped celery (about 4 large stalks)
1 large onion, chopped (about 1 cup)
1 medium green bell pepper, chopped (about 1 cup)
1 medium red bell pepper, chopped (about 1 cup)
8 ounces fresh mushrooms, cleaned and sliced
1 small package (6 ounces) frozen snow peas, slightly thawed
1 can (5 ounces) sliced water chestnuts, drained
4 medium garlic cloves, minced
¼ cup soy sauce
Generous grating black pepper

1. In a small bowl, mix ½ cup broth into cornstarch and stir until cornstarch is dissolved. Set aside.

2. Spray a large nonstick skillet generously with nonstick cooking spray and add celery, onion, green and red peppers, mushrooms, snow peas, water chestnuts and garlic. Stir-fry vegetables over high heat for 5 minutes, or until tender-crisp. (If needed, add some of the remaining 1½ cups broth, 1 tablespoon at a time, to keep vegetables from sticking.)

3. Add any remaining broth, soy sauce and pepper to vegetables. Quickly stir cornstarch mixture and add to vegetables. Cook, stirring gently, until mixture thickens and liquid becomes clear, 2 to 3 minutes. Serve immediately.

PER SERVING: CALORIES: 102; FAT: 1 G; CHOLESTEROL: 0 MG; SODIUM: 986 MG;

PROTEIN: 5 G; CARBOHYDRATE: 20 G

# Rice and Bean Medley

*Keith Van Gasken*

MAKES APPROXIMATELY 10 SERVINGS, EACH 1 CUP

"FANTASTIC" IS THE WORD one of our All-American tasters used
to describe this vegetarian delight—a filling combination of
legumes, nutty brown rice and vegetables—seasoned with
Parmesan cheese, garlic, fresh parsley and oregano. Serve as a main
dish on a bed of slightly wilted spinach or as a side dish. This makes
a large quantity and is good the next day.

    4   cups water
    1⅔  cups uncooked long-grain brown rice
    4   medium carrots, chopped (about 1½ cups)
    1   large onion, chopped (about 1 cup)
    1   medium green bell pepper, chopped (about 1 cup)
    1   large celery stalk, chopped (about ¾ cup)
    ¾   cup chopped fresh parsley
    2   cans (14 ounces each) chopped tomatoes with juice
    1   can (14 ounces) kidney beans, drained
    2   large garlic cloves, minced
    ½   cup shredded Parmesan cheese (2 ounces)
    2   teaspoons dried oregano
        Generous grating black pepper

1. To cook rice: Bring water to a boil. Add rice, stir once, then reduce heat to low. Cover and simmer for 45 to 50 minutes, or until rice
is tender but firm and water has been absorbed. (You need about 5
cups cooked rice; you may have some left over.) Remove from heat
and set aside.

2. Preheat oven to 350 degrees F. Place carrots, onion, green pepper,
celery and parsley in a large saucepan. Add ½ cup water, cover, bring
to a boil and steam just until tender-crisp, 3 to 5 minutes. Drain and
set aside.

3. In a large Dutch oven or casserole, with a wooden spoon or a rubber spatula, gently mix together tomatoes, beans, garlic, Parmesan, oregano and pepper.

4. Stir rice and vegetable mixture into bean mixture. Cover and bake for 20 minutes, or until hot in center. Serve. (Leftovers can be cooled, tightly covered and stored in casserole.)

PER SERVING: CALORIES: 200; FAT: 2.5 G; CHOLESTEROL: 3 MG; SODIUM: 399 MG; PROTEIN: 7 G; CARBOHYDRATE: 39 G

# Salads, Dressings and Relishes

# Fat-Free Creamy Italian Dressing

*Don Mauer*

MAKES ABOUT 2 CUPS OR 16 SERVINGS,
EACH 2 TABLESPOONS

D ON'S DRESSING, which can double as a salad dressing or as a vegetable dip, is a big hit with everyone who samples it. This recipe was slightly adapted from one in Don Mauer's book *Lean and Lovin' It* (Chapters Publishing).

1½ cups nonfat mayonnaise
2 tablespoons white wine vinegar
2 tablespoons lemon juice
2 tablespoons water
2 teaspoons Worcestershire sauce
2 teaspoons honey
2 large garlic cloves, minced
1 teaspoon dried oregano or 1 tablespoon fresh
1 teaspoon dried basil or 1 tablespoon fresh

In a medium mixing bowl, whisk together all ingredients until thoroughly combined. Cover tightly and refrigerate for at least 1 hour before serving. Serve cold.

PER SERVING: CALORIES: 20; FAT: 0 G; CHOLESTEROL: 0 MG; SODIUM: 201 MG; PROTEIN: 0 G; CARBOHYDRATE: 4 G

# French Bread Croutons

*Joanna M.*

MAKES ABOUT 6 CUPS OR 18 SERVINGS, EACH ⅓ CUP

MY KIDS BEG ME to serve these croutons instead of commercial high-fat types, because they make every salad special. They are also a great way to use up bread that is several days old.

Olive oil cooking spray
1    loaf (8 ounces) French or Italian bread,
     cut into cubes (about 6 cups)
     Generous sprinkling garlic powder (about 1 teaspoon)
     Generous sprinkling Italian seasoning
     (about 1 teaspoon)

1. Preheat oven to 400 degrees F, with a rack in center. Spray a jellyroll pan or a cookie sheet with nonstick cooking spray.

2. Spread bread cubes in a single layer on pan and spray with a fairly heavy, even coating of cooking spray. Sprinkle with garlic powder and Italian seasoning.

3. Bake for about 15 minutes, or until croutons are lightly browned and crisp; watch closely. Cool completely. Croutons may be stored in an airtight container at room temperature for 2 to 3 weeks.

PER SERVING: CALORIES: 37; FAT: 0.5 G; CHOLESTEROL: 0 MG; SODIUM: 77 MG; PROTEIN: 1 G; CARBOHYDRATE: 7 G

# Confetti Cabbage Salad

*Debbie T.*

SERVES 8

PERFECT FOR A PICNIC, this fat-free slaw keeps in the refrigerator for days. It goes well with low-fat hot dogs and vegetarian baked beans.

SALAD

1 bag (16 ounces) coleslaw mix or 1 pound cabbage, shredded
1 medium cucumber (9-10 ounces), chopped
1 small green bell pepper, chopped (½ cup)
1 jar (4 ounces) pimientos

DRESSING

½ cup granulated sugar
½ cup apple cider vinegar
½ cup water
1 teaspoon celery seed or mustard seed
½ teaspoon salt

1. **To make salad**: In a large nonaluminum bowl, mix ingredients and refrigerate.

2. **To make dressing**: In a medium nonaluminum saucepan, combine all ingredients and bring to a boil. Cool.

3. Toss dressing with cabbage mixture. Cover tightly. Refrigerate for at least 1 hour before serving. (The mixture will shrink as it sits.)

PER SERVING: CALORIES: 73; FAT: 0 G; CHOLESTEROL: 0 MG; SODIUM: 145 MG;
PROTEIN: 1 G; CARBOHYDRATE: 18 G

# Perfect Caesar Salad

*Joanna M.*

SERVES 6

INEVER WOULD HAVE BELIEVED I could sneak this low-fat version past my family of Caesar-salad lovers. But they adored it! It's got all the flavor but just a fraction of the fat of a traditional Caesar salad. (Note that you have to soak the garlic in olive oil overnight.)

  2   large garlic cloves, halved
  1   tablespoon olive oil
  ¼   cup egg substitute, thawed
  2   tablespoons nonfat mayonnaise
  2   tablespoons lemon juice
  2   teaspoons Dijon-style mustard
  2   teaspoons anchovy paste
  1   teaspoon Worcestershire sauce
      Generous grating black pepper
  1   large head romaine lettuce, washed,
        drained and torn into bite-sized pieces
  ¼   cup grated Parmesan or Romano cheese (1 ounce)
      Optional: French Bread Croutons (page 270)

1. At least 1 night before you plan to serve this salad, place halved garlic cloves in oil in a covered container and refrigerate.

2. When ready to prepare salad, remove 2 garlic clove halves and discard. In a small bowl, mash remaining garlic clove halves into oil and add egg substitute, mayonnaise, lemon juice, mustard, anchovy paste, Worcestershire and pepper. Blend thoroughly with a fork or a whisk.

3. In a large bowl, toss lettuce and Parmesan or Romano. Add dressing and toss lightly. Top with croutons, if desired. Serve immediately.

PER SERVING: CALORIES: 79; FAT: 5 G; CHOLESTEROL: 3 MG; SODIUM: 184 MG;
PROTEIN: 5 G; CARBOHYDRATE: 5 G

# Polynesian Carrot Salad

*JoAnna M. Lund*

SERVES 4 TO 6

ATASTY WAY TO BOOST YOUR BETA CAROTENE, this salad combines shredded carrots, fruits and coconut. It is perfect with grilled swordfish and fresh corn on the cob. (If desired, you can use ¼ teaspoon coconut flavoring in place of shredded coconut.) This recipe was adapted from one in JoAnna Lund's *HELP: Healthy Exchanges Lifetime Plan* (G.P. Putnam's Sons).

  1   pound carrots, shredded (about 3 cups)
  1   cup well-drained crushed pineapple
      (reserve 2 tablespoons juice)
  ¼   cup dark or golden raisins
  1   tablespoon shredded coconut
  ¼   cup nonfat mayonnaise
  1   tablespoon orange juice concentrate

1. In a large nonaluminum bowl, gently combine carrots, pineapple, raisins and coconut. Set aside.

2. In a small bowl, whisk together mayonnaise, reserved pineapple juice and orange juice concentrate. Toss with carrot mixture. Refrigerate until ready to serve. Serve cold.

PER SERVING: CALORIES: 87; FAT: 0.5 G; CHOLESTEROL: 0 MG; SODIUM: 114 MG; PROTEIN: 1 G; CARBOHYDRATE: 21 G

# Red Bean Salad with Corn and Onions

*Lynne C.*

MAKES 5½ TO 6 CUPS OR ABOUT 10 SERVINGS

THE SWEET-AND-SOUR COMBINATION of beans and corn nicely complements Mexican foods. A delicious alternative to everyday salads, this one is fat-free and a good source of fiber. (You could substitute chick-peas or kidney beans for the red beans.)

2 cans (15 ounces each) red beans, rinsed thoroughly
1 can (15 ounces) whole-kernel corn, drained
1 large onion, sliced
¼ cup plus 2 tablespoons red wine vinegar
2 large garlic cloves, minced
2 packets low-calorie sweetener, such as Equal,
  or more to taste
  Generous grating black pepper

1. In a large nonaluminum bowl, mix all ingredients.

2. Cover and refrigerate for several hours or overnight. Just before serving, adjust seasonings to taste. Serve cold.

PER SERVING: CALORIES: 117; FAT: 0.5 G; CHOLESTEROL: 0 MG; SODIUM: 256 MG;
PROTEIN: 6 G; CARBOHYDRATE: 24 G

# Mediterranean Rice Salad

*Ann F.*

MAKES 7 TO 8 CUPS OR ABOUT 14 SERVINGS

I LIKE THE COOL, REFRESHING TASTE of this combination as is, but you may choose to dress it with 2 ounces of crumbled feta cheese and/or a small handful of sliced black olives. (The salad has no fat, so you can splurge a little.) You can also garnish with blueberries, grapes or honeydew melon cubes or balls. To prevent gummy rice, follow package directions precisely. Avoid stirring while cooking and cool completely before adding ingredients. Don't overmix.

DRESSING
1¼ cups nonfat plain yogurt
½ cup nonfat mayonnaise
3 tablespoons lemon juice (about 1 lemon)
1 large garlic clove, minced
¼ teaspoon dried mint leaves
Generous grating black pepper
Salt to taste

SALAD
2⅔ cups water
1⅓ cups uncooked long-grain white rice
1 large celery stalk, chopped (about ¾ cup)
1 medium cucumber (9-10 ounces), cut into ¼-inch-thick slices and halved (about 1½ cups)
1 small green bell pepper, chopped (about ½ cup)
1 bunch green onions, sliced thinly (about ½ cup)
¼ cup chopped fresh parsley

1. **To make dressing:** Whisk together all ingredients in a small bowl. Set aside.

2. **To make salad:** Bring water to a boil. Add rice, stir once, then reduce heat to low. Cover and simmer for 18 to 20 minutes, or until rice is tender but firm and water is absorbed. (You will have about 4 cups of cooked rice.) Remove lid and cool completely.

3. In a large bowl, toss together celery, cucumber, green pepper, green onions and parsley.

4. Add rice and dressing and toss gently to combine. Refrigerate for at least 1 hour before serving. Serve cold.

PER SERVING: CALORIES: 80; FAT: 0 G; CHOLESTEROL: 0 MG; SODIUM: 93 MG; PROTEIN: 2 G; CARBOHYDRATE: 17 G

# Piccalilli Potato Salad

*Don C.*

MAKES ABOUT 6 CUPS OR 12 SERVINGS

TAKE THE MASTERS' LEAD and bring something you can eat when you go to social events. Don's potato salad is a great solution when you're asked to "bring a dish to pass." And no one will know it's fat-free—unless you tell them.

DRESSING
⅓  cup nonfat mayonnaise
⅓  cup nonfat plain yogurt
2  tablespoons skim milk
2  tablespoons sweet pickle juice
1  tablespoon Dijon-style mustard
½  teaspoon prepared horseradish

SALAD
2  pounds (about 7 fairly large) red-skinned potatoes, cooked, cooled and cubed
2  medium celery stalks, chopped (about 1 cup)
2  hard-cooked eggs, whites only, chopped
3  tablespoons sweet pickle relish
2  tablespoons chopped green onion (include some green tops)
1  teaspoon salt
½  teaspoon dried dill weed
   Generous grating black pepper

1. **To make dressing:** In a small bowl, whisk all ingredients together until creamy. Set aside.

2. **To make salad:** In a large mixing bowl, gently toss together all ingredients.

3. Pour dressing over salad mixture and toss gently. Adjust seasonings, if desired, and refrigerate until ready to serve. Serve cold.

PER SERVING: CALORIES: 80; FAT: 0 G; CHOLESTEROL: 0 MG; SODIUM: 318 MG; PROTEIN: 2 G; CARBOHYDRATE: 18 G

# Pesto Pasta Salad with Asparagus

*Stan J.*

MAKES 11 TO 12 CUPS OR 12 GENEROUS SERVINGS

NOTHING BEATS PESTO AND PASTA—except the pesto, pasta, asparagus and tomatoes that harmonize in this savory salad. It's a must for garlic and onion lovers and is perfect for a picnic, party or potluck supper.

### PESTO

1 cup firmly packed fresh basil leaves
2 large garlic cloves
¼ cup grated Parmesan cheese, plus
 2 tablespoons for garnish
2 tablespoons chopped walnuts (½ ounce)
2 tablespoons olive oil

### SALAD

16 ounces dried rotini pasta
2 cups cut-up (into ½-inch pieces) asparagus
 (about 1 pound, trimmed)
1 pound tomatoes, diced (about 2 cups)
1 small onion, chopped (⅓ cup)
2 tablespoons red or white wine vinegar
½ teaspoon salt
 Generous grating black pepper

1. **To make pesto:** In a blender or a food processor fitted with the metal blade, process basil, garlic, ¼ cup Parmesan, walnuts and oil until almost pureed. If mixture is too thick, add 1 to 2 teaspoons water. Set aside.

2. **To make salad:** In a large pot of boiling water, cook pasta according to package directions until tender but firm, 8 to 10 minutes. Drain. Rinse briefly with cold water. Drain again. Set aside.

3. Meanwhile, steam asparagus for 3 to 5 minutes, or until somewhat tender but still crisp. Run cold water over asparagus to stop cooking process. Drain.

4. In a large bowl, gently toss together pasta, asparagus, tomatoes, onion, vinegar, salt, pepper and reserved pesto. Just before serving, garnish with remaining 2 tablespoons Parmesan. Serve immediately or cover and chill.

PER SERVING: CALORIES: 202; FAT: 5 G; CHOLESTEROL: 0 MG; SODIUM: 139 MG;

PROTEIN: 4 G; CARBOHYDRATE: 33 G

# Pasta, Basil and Cannellini Salad

*Anna M.*

MAKES 8 TO 9 CUPS OR 10 GENEROUS SERVINGS

THIS TOMATO-BEAN COMBINATION gets its flavor from red onion, garlic, Italian seasoning, fresh basil and Parmesan cheese. Serve as a main dish with foccacia bread and melon slices or as a side dish with grilled fish or chicken.

8 ounces dried ziti pasta
1 tablespoon olive oil
1 small red onion, chopped (about ⅓ cup)
2 large garlic cloves, minced
1 can (15 ounces) cannellini beans, drained
1 can (approximately 14 ounces) diced tomatoes
  with juice (and garlic, if desired)
½ cup sliced black olives (2 ounces)
⅓ cup chopped fresh basil
⅓ cup grated Parmesan cheese (1½ ounces)
¼ cup red wine vinegar
1 teaspoon Italian seasoning

1. In a large pot of boiling water, cook pasta according to package directions until tender but firm, 10 to 12 minutes. Drain. Rinse briefly with cold water. Drain again. Set aside.

2. Heat oil in a small skillet over medium heat and sauté onion and garlic for 2 to 3 minutes, until limp but not browned. Remove from heat.

3. In a large nonaluminum bowl, gently toss together sautéed onion and garlic, pasta and remaining ingredients. Refrigerate for at least 1 hour before serving. Serve cold.

PER SERVING: CALORIES: 156; FAT: 3 G; CHOLESTEROL: 0 MG; SODIUM: 281 MG; PROTEIN: 4 G; CARBOHYDRATE: 26 G

# Fruits and Greens in Raspberry Vinaigrette

*Stan J.*

SERVES 4

SALAD GREENS AND FRUIT combine in a sweet-and-sour vinaigrette that has no fat. The salty pretzels, a nearly fat-free alternative to nuts or croutons, contrast with the dressing.

VINAIGRETTE DRESSING
6 tablespoons raspberry wine vinegar
3 tablespoons granulated sugar
1½ teaspoons Dijon-style mustard
1½ teaspoons chopped fresh chives
Salt and freshly ground black pepper

SALAD
1 bag (10 ounces) mixed greens
(romaine, leaf lettuce, spinach)
1½ cups melon balls (cantaloupe and/or honeydew melon)
½ pint fresh raspberries (1 heaping cup)
⅓ cup fresh blueberries
½ cup broken pretzels (about 1 ounce)

1. **To make dressing:** Place all ingredients in a small jar or plastic container with a tight-fitting lid. Shake until well blended, about 1 minute. Refrigerate until needed.

2. **To make salad:** Place greens and fruit in a large bowl. Shake dressing well and pour over; toss gently until combined. Serve immediately. Top individual servings with pretzels.

PER SERVING: CALORIES: 125; FAT: 1 G; CHOLESTEROL: 0 MG; SODIUM: 190 MG;

PROTEIN: 3 G; CARBOHYDRATE: 29 G

# Raisin Waldorf Salad

*Beth W.*

MAKES ABOUT 7 CUPS OR 10 SERVINGS

BETH DEEMS THIS CRUNCHY, FRUITY COMBINATION her favorite recipe. She likes to use Braeburn apples from Australia—they are a firm, crunchy apple available most of the year. If you like more zing, try using a tart apple, such as Granny Smith.

SALAD

5   firm medium apples (about 1½ pounds),
    cored and cut into ½-inch cubes
3   medium celery stalks, thinly sliced (1½ cups)
8   ounces juice-packed pineapple tidbits, well drained
⅓   cup dark raisins
2   tablespoons unsalted sunflower seeds

DRESSING

1   container (6 ounces) nonfat orange or lemon yogurt
1   tablespoon nonfat mayonnaise
1   teaspoon honey

1. **To make salad**: In a large bowl, gently mix salad ingredients.

2. **To make dressing**: In a small bowl, whisk together yogurt, mayonnaise and honey. Pour over salad and toss gently. Serve immediately or cover and chill.

PER SERVING: CALORIES: 94; FAT: 1 G; CHOLESTEROL: 0 MG; SODIUM: 37 MG; PROTEIN: 2 G; CARBOHYDRATE: 21 G

# Cranberry-Orange Relish

*Irene H.*

MAKES 3 TO 3½ CUPS OR 6 SERVINGS

ALTHOUGH FRESH CRANBERRIES are seasonal, you can buy a few extra bags for the freezer and make this pretty relish year-round. This light version has a fraction of the sugar of the traditional relish, which often contains as much as two cups.

1   bag (12 ounces) fresh cranberries
1   small orange (about 5 ounces)
1   medium apple (about 5 ounces),
     preferably Granny Smith, cored
¼   cup granulated sugar
3   packets Sweet 'N Low
     Dash salt

1. Wash cranberries, orange and apple. Quarter orange and apple and remove seeds.

2. Place cranberries, orange quarters (including rind) and apple quarters in a food processor fitted with the metal blade. Process until chopped to desired consistency. (You can also use a hand grinder.)

3. Pour cranberry mixture into a medium bowl and stir in sugar, sweetener and salt. Refrigerate for at least 1 hour before serving. Serve cold.

PER SERVING: CALORIES: 84; FAT: 0 G; CHOLESTEROL: 0 MG; SODIUM: 18 MG; PROTEIN: 0 G; CARBOHYDRATE: 22 G

# Side Dishes

# Carrots in Orange Sauce

### Keith Van Gasken

#### SERVES 4 GENEROUSLY

K EITH'S ORANGE-HONEY GLAZE is simple yet jazzes up carrots without adding any fat. This makes a wonderful accompaniment to a holiday dinner of roast turkey, beef or pork.

1 pound baby carrots, peeled
1 teaspoon cornstarch
½ cup orange juice
2 tablespoons honey
⅛ teaspoon ground cinnamon
⅛ teaspoon ground nutmeg
¼ teaspoon salt
2 tablespoons chopped fresh parsley

1. Steam carrots until tender but still crisp, about 10 minutes. Drain well; cover to keep warm.

2. In a medium nonaluminum saucepan, with a wire whisk, combine cornstarch, orange juice, honey, cinnamon, nutmeg and salt. Cook, uncovered, over medium-high heat, stirring often, until mixture comes to a boil and is translucent. Lower heat and continue cooking, stirring constantly, for 1 more minute. Remove from heat and pour over carrots. Garnish with parsley and serve.

PER SERVING: CALORIES: 89; FAT: 0.5 G; CHOLESTEROL: 0 MG; SODIUM: 172 MG;

PROTEIN: 1 G; CARBOHYDRATE: 21 G

# Danish Cabbage

*Keith Van Gasken*

SERVES 6

THIS SWEET-AND-SOUR MEDLEY of red cabbage, apples and onion makes a nice accompaniment to a ham or pork main dish. It can be made ahead and reheated in the oven or microwave.

¾ pound red cabbage, cored and shredded
3 tart medium apples (about 1 pound),
  such as Granny Smith, cored and diced
1 medium onion, chopped (about ⅔ cup)
¼ cup water
2 tablespoons red wine vinegar
2 tablespoons granulated sugar
¼ teaspoon salt
⅛ teaspoon ground allspice

1. Place all ingredients in a large nonaluminum pot, cover and bring to a boil over medium-high heat. Stir occasionally to prevent sticking.

2. Reduce heat to low and simmer, covered, for 30 minutes, or until tender. Stir occasionally. Adjust seasonings to taste and serve.

PER SERVING: CALORIES: 76; FAT: 0 G; CHOLESTEROL: 0 MG; SODIUM: 95 MG; PROTEIN: 1 G; CARBOHYDRATE: 19 G

# Cabbage and Apples with Swiss Cheese

*Beth W.*

SERVES 8

THIS DISH MAKES A GOOD GO-ALONG for roast pork or turkey. The combination of cabbage, Swiss cheese, apples and nonfat sour cream is delicious. (This dish can be made ahead and reheated.) Serve any leftovers for lunch.

- ¼ cup water
- 1 pound cabbage, coarsely chopped (about 7 cups)
- 1 medium onion, chopped (about ⅔ cup)
- ¼ teaspoon celery seed
- ¼ teaspoon salt
- ¼ teaspoon freshly ground black pepper
- 2 medium apples, cored and chopped into ¾-inch chunks (2½ cups)
- 1 teaspoon granulated sugar
- 1½ cups shredded reduced-fat Swiss cheese (6 ounces)
- 3 tablespoons nonfat sour cream

1. In a large pot, combine water, cabbage, onion, celery seed, salt and pepper. Cover and cook over medium heat, stirring occasionally, for 7 to 10 minutes, or until vegetables begin to soften.

2. Add apples and sugar, cover and cook for 5 minutes more, or until apples just begin to soften. Remove from heat and stir in 1 cup cheese and sour cream. Place in a serving dish, sprinkle with remaining ½ cup cheese and serve.

PER SERVING: CALORIES: 99; FAT: 4 G; CHOLESTEROL: 12 MG; SODIUM: 182 MG; PROTEIN: 6 G; CARBOHYDRATE: 11 G

# Corn Custard Casserole

*Paul R.*

SERVES 10 AS A SIDE DISH

THIS CREAMY CUSTARD—a blend of corn, creamed corn, egg whites and nonfat sour cream—is thickened with corn-muffin mix and gets some punch from mild green chilies. It makes a great accompaniment to Mexican foods. To serve as a main dish, offer larger portions garnished with strips of red and green bell pepper.

1   can (15 ounces) corn, drained
1   can (15 ounces) creamed corn
1   can (4.5 ounces) chopped mild green chilies, drained
1   tablespoon minced fresh onion
1   box (8.5 ounces) Jiffy Corn Muffin Mix
4   large egg whites
1   cup nonfat sour cream
4   tablespoons diet margarine, melted

1. Preheat oven to 350 degrees F. Spray an 8-x-10-inch pan with non-stick cooking spray and set aside.

2. In a large bowl, mix all ingredients until well combined.

3. Pour into prepared pan and bake for 1 hour, or until edges pull away from sides of pan and custard is set in center. Serve promptly.

PER SERVING: CALORIES: 219; FAT: 6 G; CHOLESTEROL: 0 MG; SODIUM: 764 MG; PROTEIN: 7 G; CARBOHYDRATE: 38 G

# Spinach-Broccoli Casserole

*Jennie C.*

SERVES 8 AS A SIDE DISH

CUSTARD LOVERS will adore this rich-tasting casserole of spinach, broccoli, creamy soup, eggs and cheese. The dish can accompany broiled or grilled seafood or chicken. For a complete meal, add a grated-carrot salad. Larger portions can be served as a vegetarian main dish. Leftovers are good for lunch.

1 package (10 ounces) frozen chopped spinach, thawed and drained
1 package (10 ounces) frozen chopped broccoli, thawed and drained
1 can (10¾ ounces) Campbell's Healthy Request Cream of Broccoli Soup
3 large eggs, beaten with whisk
½ cup shredded Parmesan cheese (2 ounces)
⅓ cup nonfat mayonnaise

1. Preheat oven to 325 degrees F. Spray a 2-quart baking dish with nonstick cooking spray. Set aside.

2. In a large bowl, mix spinach, broccoli, soup, eggs, Parmesan and mayonnaise with a large spoon or rubber spatula until thoroughly combined. Pour into baking dish.

3. Place baking dish in a larger baking dish and pour hot water into pan to reach halfway up outside of smaller dish. Bake, uncovered, for 1 hour, or until a knife inserted in center comes out clean. Serve promptly.

PER SERVING: CALORIES: 93; FAT: 4 G; CHOLESTEROL: 85 MG; SODIUM: 391 MG; PROTEIN: 7 G; CARBOHYDRATE: 8 G

# Eggplant Soufflé

*Harriet P.*

SERVES 4 AS A MAIN DISH OR 6 AS A SIDE DISH

HARRIET'S SOUFFLÉ is an unassuming puff of steamed eggplant, eggs and bread crumbs, accented with chopped green onion and basil. It can be served as either a side dish or a main dish with a citrus salad. Instead of baking it, you can drop the eggplant mixture by spoonfuls onto a hot griddle or skillet and brown like potato pancakes.

1   large eggplant (about 1¼ pounds),
     peeled and cut into ½-inch cubes
2   large eggs, separated
½   cup skim milk
¾   cup bread crumbs
1   large green onion, chopped
¾   teaspoon dried basil
½   teaspoon salt
     Generous grating black pepper

1. Preheat oven to 350 degrees F. Place eggplant in a medium saucepan; add about 1 inch water. Bring to a boil over medium-high heat, cover and reduce heat to low. Simmer for 7 to 10 minutes, or until eggplant is soft. Drain and mash thoroughly with a fork. Set aside.

2. Spray a 1-quart casserole or soufflé dish with nonstick cooking spray, preferably olive-oil-flavored. Set aside.

3. In a large bowl, with an electric mixer, beat egg whites until soft peaks form. Set aside. In a medium bowl, with a fork, mix mashed eggplant, egg yolks, milk, bread crumbs, green onion, basil, salt and pepper. Gently fold eggplant mixture into egg whites. Turn into prepared casserole or soufflé dish.

4. Place casserole or soufflé dish in a larger baking pan and pour hot water into pan to a depth of 1 inch. Bake, uncovered, for 35 to 40 minutes, or until a knife inserted in center comes out clean. Serve immediately.

PER SIDE-DISH SERVING: CALORIES: 107; FAT: 2.5 G; CHOLESTEROL: 71 MG;

SODIUM: 329 MG; PROTEIN: 5 G; CARBOHYDRATE: 16 G

# Sweet Potato Puff

*Keith Van Gasken*

A UNIQUE SWEET POTATO SOUFFLÉ, this dish relies on banana for its sweetening power. It makes great leftovers too. Serve with roast turkey, chicken or pork and a low-fat slaw.

1 large egg, separated
2 cups cooked and mashed sweet potatoes
   (about 2 pounds unpeeled raw or 18 ounces
   canned unsweetened)
1 cup mashed very ripe banana (about 2 medium,
   11-12 ounces before peeling)
½ tablespoon Butter Buds Sprinkles
½ teaspoon salt
⅛ teaspoon ground nutmeg

1. Preheat oven to 350 degrees F. Spray a 1-quart baking dish with nonstick cooking spray. Set aside.

2. In a small mixing bowl, with an electric mixer, beat egg white until stiff peaks form. Set aside.

3. In a large bowl, with electric mixer on medium speed, whip sweet potatoes, banana, egg yolk, Butter Buds, salt and nutmeg until smooth, about 2 minutes.

4. Gently fold in whipped egg white. Spread evenly in prepared dish and bake for 35 to 45 minutes, or until a knife inserted in center comes out clean. Serve immediately.

PER SERVING: CALORIES: 243; FAT: 2 G; CHOLESTEROL: 53 MG; SODIUM: 331 MG; PROTEIN: 5 G; CARBOHYDRATE: 53 G

# Scalloped Onions with Canadian Bacon

*Joy C.*

SERVES 6

THIS CREAMY COMBINATION of onions, eggs, milk and smoky Canadian bacon is especially tasty. The leftovers are delicious warmed in the microwave.

⅔ cup skim milk
½ cup evaporated skim milk
2 tablespoons all-purpose flour
¼ cup thawed egg substitute or 1 large egg, beaten
5 medium onions (about 20 ounces total), thinly sliced
⅓ cup shredded Parmesan cheese (1½ ounces)
2 ounces thinly sliced Canadian-style bacon,
 chopped into ½-inch pieces

1. Preheat oven to 350 degrees F. Spray a 1½-quart casserole with non-stick cooking spray. Set aside.

2. In a small mixing bowl, slowly whisk skim and evaporated milk into flour until no lumps remain. Mix in egg substitute or egg; set aside.

3. Spread half of sliced onions over bottom of casserole. Sprinkle evenly with half of Parmesan and half of bacon. Top with remaining onions, Parmesan and bacon. Stir milk mixture and pour over ingredients in casserole.

4. Bake, uncovered, for 30 to 40 minutes, or until onions are tender and casserole is piping hot in center. Serve promptly.

PER SERVING: CALORIES: 113; FAT: 2.5 G; CHOLESTEROL: 9 MG; SODIUM: 267 MG; PROTEIN: 9 G; CARBOHYDRATE: 14 G

# Creole Beans

*Diane J.*

SERVES 8 TO 10 GENEROUSLY

THESE LIVELY-TASTING LIMAS makes a nice alternative to tradi-tional pork and beans at summer picnics.

1 tablespoon bacon fat or vegetable oil
1 large onion, chopped (about 1 cup)
1 medium green bell pepper, chopped (about 1 cup)
1 medium celery stalk, sliced (about ½ cup)
2 large garlic cloves, minced
1 tablespoon all-purpose flour
Generous grating black pepper
2 cans (15 ounces each) stewed tomatoes, with juice
¼ cup chili sauce
2 teaspoons prepared mustard
1 teaspoon Worcestershire sauce
1 tablespoon light or dark brown sugar
2 cans (15 ounces each) lima beans, rinsed and drained, or 3½ cups frozen lima beans, cooked according to package directions and drained
2 slices bacon, cooked crisp and crumbled

1. In a large nonstick skillet, heat bacon fat or oil over medium-high heat. Add onion, green pepper, celery and garlic and sauté until soft, 5 to 7 minutes. Stir in flour and pepper.

2. Reduce heat to medium and add tomatoes, chili sauce, mustard, Worcestershire and brown sugar. Simmer for 2 minutes.

3. Gently mix in lima beans and heat through for 1 to 2 minutes. Just before serving, sprinkle with bacon. Serve hot.

PER SERVING: CALORIES: 125; FAT: 2.5 G; CHOLESTEROL: 0 MG; SODIUM: 406 MG; PROTEIN: 6 G; CARBOHYDRATE: 22 G

# Green Bean-Almond Rice

*Diane J.*

SERVES 6

BROWN RICE, GREEN BEANS AND RED PEPPER team up in this nutty, crunchy blend that complements lean meat dishes.

2½   cups water
1    teaspoon beef bouillon granules
1    cup uncooked long-grain brown rice
1    tablespoon margarine or butter
⅓    cup slivered almonds
½    cup chopped onion (½ a large onion)
1    small red bell pepper, chopped (about ½ cup)
1    package (9-10 ounces) frozen French-style
     green beans, thawed
½    teaspoon salt
     Generous grating black pepper
¼    teaspoon dried tarragon

1. Bring water to a boil, add bouillon and stir until dissolved. Add rice, stir once; reduce heat to low. Cover and simmer for 45 to 50 minutes, or until rice is tender but firm and water is absorbed. (You will have about 3 cups cooked rice.) Remove from heat and set aside.

2. Melt margarine or butter in a large nonstick skillet over medium-high heat. Add almonds and sauté until lightly browned, 2 to 3 minutes.

3. Add onion and red pepper and cook for 2 minutes, or until just tender. Add rice, green beans, salt, pepper and tarragon. Cook, tossing gently, until heated through, 4 to 5 minutes. Serve immediately.

PER SERVING: CALORIES: 186; FAT: 6 G; CHOLESTEROL: 0 MG; SODIUM: 377 MG; PROTEIN: 5 G; CARBOHYDRATE: 29 G

# Gingered Rice with Sweet Potatoes

*Marie C.*

SERVES 6

SWEET POTATOES, ginger and nutmeg bring home the taste of autumn in this simple, appealing rice dish. If you like, garnish it with pineapple rings. In place of white rice, try brown. It is great with ham or poultry.

| | |
|---|---|
| 1 | pound sweet potatoes (about 3 medium) |
| 1⅓ | cups water |
| ⅔ | cup uncooked long-grain white rice |
| 2 | tablespoons light or dark brown sugar |
| ½ | teaspoon ground ginger |
| ¼ | teaspoon ground nutmeg |

1. Preheat oven to 375 degrees F. Prick potatoes twice with a fork. Place in oven on a sheet of foil. Bake for 1 hour, or until soft in center when a sharp knife is inserted. When cool enough to handle, peel potatoes and cut into ½-inch cubes. Set aside.

2. Meanwhile, bring water to a boil. Add rice, stir once, then reduce heat to low. Cover and simmer for 18 to 20 minutes, or until rice is tender but firm and water is absorbed. (You will have 2 cups cooked rice.) Remove from heat and set aside.

3. In a large bowl, gently toss sweet potatoes with brown sugar, ginger and nutmeg.

4. Gently mix in rice and serve immediately.

PER SERVING: CALORIES: 139; FAT: 0 G; CHOLESTEROL: 0 MG; SODIUM: 7 MG; PROTEIN: 2 G; CARBOHYDRATE: 32 G

# Mike's French Fries

*Michael F.*

SERVES 4

M Y KIDS CALL THESE EASY-TO-DO FRIES "awesome" and "totally tubular." They are good with Cheddar Fish (page 224) or Oven-Fried Chicken (page 212).

4   large baking potatoes (about 1½ pounds), washed
1   tablespoon reduced-fat margarine
¼   teaspoon salt, or more to taste
    Freshly ground black pepper, or more to taste

1. Spray an 8-x-8-inch glass pan (2-quart) with nonstick cooking spray. Set aside.

2. Peel potatoes, if desired. Cut them into strips about ½ inch wide.

3. Place potato strips in pan and cover with plastic wrap. Vent corner or cut a few small slits in cover. Microwave potatoes on high power, rotating pan once, until they begin to get soft when pricked with a fork or a toothpick, about 7 minutes.

4. Grease a large nonstick pan with margarine. Heat over medium-high heat, add potatoes, sprinkle with salt and pepper, and fry until golden brown, 12 to 15 minutes. Just before serving, adjust seasonings, adding more salt and pepper as needed. Serve hot.

PER SERVING (UNPEELED): CALORIES: 233; FAT: 1.5 G; CHOLESTEROL: 0 MG;

SODIUM: 184 MG; PROTEIN: 5 G; CARBOHYDRATE: 51 G

# Cheesy Spuds

*Diane J.*

SERVES 4 AS A SIDE DISH OR 2 AS A MAIN DISH

THESE TWICE-BAKED POTATOES, made with nonfat sour cream, reduced-fat Cheddar cheese and fresh chives, get a new spin from basil and mushrooms. "Good flavor, good texture, just plain good," said someone who tried them for the first time. These potatoes can be served as either a main dish or a side dish.

2   very large baking potatoes (8 ounces each)
1   cup steamed chopped mushrooms
⅓   cup shredded reduced-fat sharp Cheddar cheese
    (1½ ounces)
4   tablespoons nonfat sour cream
¼   cup skim milk
1   teaspoon basil
¼   teaspoon garlic powder
¼   teaspoon salt
2   tablespoons chopped fresh chives

1. Scrub potatoes and prick each with a fork twice. Place them side by side on a paper towel in center of microwave oven. Microwave on high power for 5 to 8 minutes, or until soft in middle when poked with a sharp knife. (To bake, preheat oven to 425 degrees F, and bake for 40 to 60 minutes, or until soft.) Set aside.

2. In a medium bowl, with a fork or a whisk, blend mushrooms, Cheddar cheese, sour cream, milk, basil, garlic powder and salt. (If you plan to bake potatoes in oven, add chives now.) Set aside.

3. Scoop potato pulp from shells, leaving a ¼-inch border, and place in a shallow bowl. Pour sour-cream mixture over potato and mash together thoroughly with a fork.

4. Spoon mixture back into potato shells and sprinkle with chives. Microwave on high power for 4 to 5 minutes, or until heated through. Or bake in a 350-degree oven for about 20 minutes. Serve hot.

PER SIDE DISH SERVING (WITH SKIN): CALORIES: 170; FAT: 2 G; CHOLESTEROL: 6 MG; SODIUM: 220 MG; PROTEIN: 7 G; CARBOHYDRATE: 31 G

# Rosemary-Dijon New Potatoes

*Cathy B.*

SERVES 6

THESE SAVORY POTATOES are roasted in a sauce of Dijon mustard and olive oil and are crowned with a sprig of rosemary. They are a perfect accompaniment to a dinner of grilled salmon and steamed broccoli.

9    small or medium uniformly sized new potatoes
     (about 1½ pounds)
1    tablespoon olive oil
1    teaspoon Dijon-style mustard
½    teaspoon chicken bouillon granules
½    teaspoon salt
     Generous grating black pepper
1    package fresh rosemary (18 sections, each 1 inch long)
     or 1 tablespoon dried

1. Preheat oven to 350 degrees F. Spray an 8-x-11-inch baking dish with nonstick cooking spray. Set aside.

2. Wash and dry potatoes. Slice them in half. Make a V-cut notch (about ¼ inch deep) across entire length of rounded side of each potato half. Place potatoes in baking dish, flat side down. Set aside.

3. In a small bowl, stir together oil, mustard, bouillon, salt and pepper. Spread about ¼ teaspoon of mixture in notch of each potato half.

4. Insert a 1-inch section of rosemary or a tiny pinch of dried in each notch.

5. Cover with foil and bake for 30 minutes. Uncover and bake for 15 minutes more, or until a fork comes out easily when potatoes are pricked in center. Just before serving, spoon any pan drippings over potatoes.

PER SERVING: CALORIES: 121; FAT: 2.5 G; CHOLESTEROL: 0 MG; SODIUM: 287 MG;

PROTEIN: 2 G; CARBOHYDRATE: 23 G

# Sweets

SWEETS

# Apple Crumb Dessert

*Harriet P.*

SERVES 4

ꙅO SIMPLE, YET SO GOOD. This is the first fat-free apple crisp recipe I've enjoyed.

4   medium (about 1¼ pounds) baking apples,
    such as Granny Smith, peeled and thinly sliced
½   cup uncooked quick-cooking oatmeal
¼   cup light or dark brown sugar
2   teaspoons ground cinnamon
⅓   cup apple juice

1. Preheat oven to 350 degrees F, with a rack in center. Spray a 1-quart (9-x-9-inch) baking dish with nonstick cooking spray.

2. Spread apple slices evenly over bottom of baking dish; set aside.

3. In a small bowl, with a fork, blend together oatmeal, brown sugar and cinnamon until well mixed. Spread evenly over apples.

4. Sprinkle apple juice over top. Cover and bake for 20 to 30 minutes, or until apples are just starting to soften. Uncover and bake for 15 to 20 minutes more, or until apples are soft.

PER SERVING: CALORIES: 156; FAT: 1 G; CHOLESTEROL: 0 MG; SODIUM: 105 MG; PROTEIN: 2 G; CARBOHYDRATE: 37 G

# Fruity Bread Pudding

*Marie C.*

SERVES 6 TO 8

IN THIS UPDATE OF A CLASSIC COMFORT FOOD, chunks of white bread are soaked in maple syrup with milk and cinnamon, sprinkled with raisins, then drizzled with melted raspberry preserves. Serve as a dessert or for a special Sunday-morning breakfast.

½ cup maple syrup
1 small loaf (8 ounces) French or Italian bread (day-old), cut into 1-inch cubes
⅓ cup dark raisins
3 large eggs
1 cup skim milk
¾ cup evaporated skim milk
2 teaspoons vanilla extract
1 teaspoon ground cinnamon
⅓ cup raspberry preserves

1. Preheat oven to 325 degrees F, with a rack in center. Spray a 7-x-11-inch baking pan with nonstick cooking spray.

2. Pour maple syrup into baking pan. Distribute bread cubes evenly over maple syrup. Sprinkle with raisins. Set aside.

3. In a medium bowl, with a whisk or an eggbeater, thoroughly beat together eggs, skim milk, evaporated milk, vanilla and cinnamon. Pour evenly over bread. Refrigerate and let sit for 15 to 20 minutes, until bread has absorbed milk.

4. In a small saucepan, over low heat (or in a microwave), melt raspberry preserves. Just before baking, drizzle preserves over bread.

5. Cover with foil and bake for 15 minutes; uncover and bake for 15 to 20 minutes more, or until a knife inserted in center comes out clean and pudding is piping hot. Cool for 20 minutes before serving, or chill if you don't serve promptly. Serve warm, cold or at room temperature. Cover any leftovers tightly and refrigerate.

PER SERVING: CALORIES: 241; FAT: 3 G; CHOLESTEROL: 81 MG; SODIUM: 248 MG; PROTEIN: 8 G; CARBOHYDRATE: 46 G

# Heavenly Brownies

*Don Mauer*

MAKES 18 BROWNIES

T HESE BROWNIES ARE SO UNBELIEVABLY GOOD that it's hard to believe they have a mere 2 grams of fat apiece. The moisture comes mainly from applesauce, used in place of oil. One of the kids who tasted these described them as "heavenly." If you like, top this with Rich Chocolate Frosting (page 310). This recipe was adapted from one in Don Mauer's *Lean and Lovin' It* (Chapters Publishing).

| | |
|---|---|
| 1 | cup all-purpose flour |
| ¾ | cup unsweetened cocoa powder |
| ½ | teaspoon baking powder |
| ¼ | teaspoon salt |
| 1 | cup unsweetened plain applesauce |
| 1 | large egg |
| 6 | large egg whites |
| 2 | teaspoons vanilla extract |
| 2 | cups granulated sugar |
| 3 | tablespoons finely chopped pecans (about 1 ounce) |

1. Preheat oven to 350 degrees F, with a rack in center. Lightly spray sides and bottom of 9-x-13-inch baking pan with nonstick cooking spray. Set aside.

2. Sift together flour, cocoa powder, baking powder and salt. Set aside.

3. In a large mixing bowl, whisk together applesauce, egg, egg whites and vanilla until thoroughly combined. Add sugar and whisk until sugar is dissolved. Add dry ingredients and whisk until just moistened, 20 to 25 seconds. Do not overmix, or brownies will be tough and rubbery.

4. Pour batter evenly into prepared pan and sprinkle pecans over top.
Bake for 30 to 35 minutes, or until brownies pull away from sides of
pan. Cool. Cut into 18 squares. Store in pan, tightly covered with foil.
(Refrigerate if not eating within 1 to 2 days.)

PER BROWNIE: CALORIES: 147; FAT: 2 G; CHOLESTEROL: 12 MG; SODIUM: 66 MG;

PROTEIN: 3 G; CARBOHYDRATE: 32 G

# Rich Chocolate Frosting

*Don Mauer*

MAKES ABOUT 2 CUPS
OR 8 SERVINGS, EACH ¼ CUP;
FROSTS A 9-X-13-INCH PAN OF BROWNIES OR CAKE

THIS DELECTABLE NEARLY FAT-FREE FROSTING is perfect for low-fat brownies, cakes and cookies. This recipe was adapted from one in Don Mauer's *Lean and Lovin' It* (Chapters Publishing).

¼ cup Promise Ultra Fat Free margarine
½ cup unsweetened cocoa powder
1 tablespoon skim milk
¾ teaspoon vanilla extract
1¾ cups powdered sugar

1. In a small mixing bowl, with an electric mixer on medium speed, cream together margarine and cocoa powder. Add milk and vanilla, and mix on low speed until well blended.

2. With mixer on medium speed, add half of powdered sugar. Mix until smooth. Repeat with remaining sugar. Cover and refrigerate if not using immediately.

PER SERVING: CALORIES: 119; FAT: 1 G; CHOLESTEROL: 0 MG; SODIUM: 48 MG; PROTEIN: 1 G; CARBOHYDRATE: 29 G

# Crusty Peach Crisp

*Ann F.*

SERVES 8

MY NEIGHBOR DESCRIBED THIS CRUST-TOPPED DESSERT succinctly: "Super! It's hard to believe it's low-fat." It is scrump-
tious as is or served warm with a little fat-free vanilla ice cream
or frozen yogurt. It also makes a great breakfast treat with some cottage cheese.

½   cup light or dark brown sugar
½   cup unsweetened applesauce
1   tablespoon cornstarch
¼   teaspoon ground cinnamon
3   pounds fresh peaches or nectarines, pitted,
      peeled, if desired, and sliced
¾   cup graham cracker crumbs (from about 5 crackers)
½   cup Grape-Nuts cereal

1. Preheat oven to 350 degrees F, with a rack in center. Spray a 9-x-
9-inch baking dish with nonstick cooking spray; set aside.

2. In a large bowl, whisk together brown sugar, applesauce, cornstarch
and cinnamon until no lumps remain. Gently stir in peaches or nectarines until they are well coated. Pour into prepared pan.

3. In a small bowl, mix cracker crumbs and Grape-Nuts. Sprinkle
evenly over peaches.

4. Cover and bake for 20 minutes; uncover and bake for 20 minutes
more, or until fruit is soft when pierced with a fork and juices are bubbling. Serve warm, cold or at room temperature.

PER SERVING: CALORIES: 163; FAT: 1 G; CHOLESTEROL: 0 MG; SODIUM: 106 MG;
PROTEIN: 2 G; CARBOHYDRATE: 38 G

# Molasses-Fruit Bars

*Lois A.*

MAKES 18 BARS

WHO NEEDS STORE-BOUGHT FIG BARS when you can make these moist fruit bars in no time? They're good for dessert or breakfast.

½   cup chopped pitted dates (about 2½ ounces)
½   cup chopped pitted prunes (about 3 ounces)
½   cup dark raisins (about 3 ounces)
¼   cup molasses
¾   cup water
4   tablespoons (½ stick) margarine or butter
1   cup all-purpose flour
1   teaspoon baking soda
½   teaspoon ground cinnamon
¼   teaspoon ground nutmeg
¼   cup chopped walnuts
2   large eggs, slightly beaten
2   teaspoons vanilla extract

1. Preheat oven to 350 degrees F, with a rack in center. Spray an 8-x-11-inch baking pan with nonstick cooking spray; set aside.

2. In a large saucepan, over medium heat, bring dates, prunes, raisins, molasses and water to a boil. Stir in margarine or butter and set aside to cool.

3. In a small bowl, stir together flour, baking soda, cinnamon, nutmeg and walnuts. Set aside.

4. After fruit mixture has cooled, with a large spoon, stir in eggs and vanilla, mixing until thoroughly combined. Add dry ingredients and stir just until mixed. Pour into prepared pan and bake for 15 to 20 minutes, or until a toothpick inserted in center comes out clean. Cool. Cut into 18 bars. Store in pan, tightly covered with foil. (Refrigerate if not eating within 1 to 2 days.)

PER BAR: CALORIES: 121; FAT: 4 G; CHOLESTEROL: 24 MG; SODIUM: 110 MG; PROTEIN: 2 G; CARBOHYDRATE: 20 G

# Raisin, Date and Apple Cookies

*Lois A.*

MAKES 24 COOKIES

YOUR SWEET TOOTH will say "more" to these soft, fruity cookies, which are super for the picnic basket or lunch box. They are delicious plain or with the simple maple glaze, which adds just 10 calories (and no fat) per cookie. (The recipe calls for imitation butter flavor, which can be purchased in the supermarket spice section, near other flavorings, such as vanilla.)

### COOKIES
1 cup raisins (about 6 ounces)
½ cup chopped pitted dates (about 2½ ounces)
½ cup chopped peeled apple
1 cup water
4 tablespoons (½ stick) margarine or butter
¼ cup granulated sugar
1 teaspoon vanilla extract
¼ teaspoon imitation butter flavor
1 cup all-purpose flour
1½ teaspoons ground cinnamon
1 teaspoon baking soda

### OPTIONAL MAPLE GLAZE
½ cup powdered sugar
½-¾ tablespoon skim milk
¼ teaspoon maple flavoring
⅛ teaspoon ground cinnamon
⅛ teaspoon ground nutmeg

1. **To make cookies:** Preheat oven to 375 degrees F, with a rack in center. Spray a cookie sheet with nonstick cooking spray. Set aside.

2. In a medium saucepan, over medium-high heat, bring raisins, dates, apple and water to a boil. Simmer, uncovered, for 5 minutes to soften fruit.

3. Remove from heat and stir in margarine or butter, sugar, vanilla and butter flavoring. Stir until margarine or butter is melted. Set aside to cool for 15 minutes.

4. In a small bowl, stir together flour, cinnamon and baking soda. Add to fruit mixture and stir until well blended.

5. Drop dough by tablespoonfuls about 2 inches apart onto prepared cookie sheet. Bake for 10 minutes, or until a toothpick inserted in cookies comes out clean. Remove from pan immediately and cool on a wire rack. Store in an airtight container. (Refrigerate if not eating within 2 to 3 days.)

6. **To make optional glaze:** In a small bowl, stir together powdered sugar, milk, maple flavoring, cinnamon and nutmeg.

7. Spread slightly rounded quarter-teaspoonfuls of glaze on cooled cookies. Serve immediately.

PER COOKIE WITHOUT GLAZE: CALORIES: 77; FAT: 2 G; CHOLESTEROL: 0 MG; SODIUM: 76 MG; PROTEIN: 1 G; CARBOHYDRATE: 15 G

PER COOKIE WITH GLAZE: CALORIES: 87; FAT: 2 G; CHOLESTEROL: 0 MG; SODIUM: 76 MG; PROTEIN: 1 G; CARBOHYDRATE: 17 G

# Crispy Golden Macaroons

*Evelyn C.*

MAKES APPROXIMATELY 20 COOKIES

EVELYN MARKEDLY LOWERED THE FAT in this traditional favorite by adding two different kinds of cereal and substituting low-fat condensed milk for the regular version. At holiday time, stick a candied cherry in the center of each cookie.

⅔ cup low-fat sweetened condensed milk
1 cup corn flakes cereal
1 cup crisp rice cereal
¾ cup shredded sweetened coconut

1. Preheat oven to 375 degrees F, with a rack in center. Spray a cookie sheet with nonstick cooking spray. Set aside.

2. In a large bowl, thoroughly combine all ingredients with a wooden spoon or rubber spatula. Drop mixture from a tablespoon in walnut-sized mounds 2 inches apart onto prepared cookie sheet.

3. Bake for 8 to 10 minutes, or until cookies start to turn golden brown. Remove cookies from sheet after 1 minute of cooling and cool completely on a wire rack. Store in an airtight container. (Refrigerate if not eating within 2 to 3 days.)

PER COOKIE: CALORIES: 57; FAT: 1 G; CHOLESTEROL: 0 MG; SODIUM: 44 MG; PROTEIN: 1 G; CARBOHYDRATE: 10 G

# Orange Delight Pound Cake

*Patsy K.*

SERVES 10

THIS MOIST, RICH CAKE tastes as if it is loaded with oil and sour cream, but it has just 3 grams of fat per serving. It is delectable plain but is also good with Tropical Fruit Sauce (page 334) or with cold mandarin orange slices for garnish.

1 package reduced-fat yellow cake mix
⅔ cup nonfat plain yogurt
½ cup thawed orange juice concentrate
½ cup water
3 large egg whites

1. Preheat oven to 350 degrees F, with a rack in center. Spray a 10-inch Bundt pan or angel food cake pan with nonstick cooking spray. Set aside.

2. In a large mixing bowl, with an electric mixer on low speed, mix cake mix, yogurt, orange juice concentrate, water and egg whites until thoroughly blended. Turn mixer to high speed and beat for 5 minutes.

3. Pour batter into prepared pan and bake for 35 to 40 minutes, or until a toothpick inserted in center comes out clean. Let stand for 10 minutes, then turn upside down on a wire rack. Cool for 20 to 30 minutes; run a knife around edges to loosen sides and remove from pan. Cool completely on rack before serving.

PER SERVING: CALORIES: 230; FAT: 3 G; CHOLESTEROL: 0 MG; SODIUM: 365 MG; PROTEIN: 4 G; CARBOHYDRATE: 47 G

# Chocolate Upside-Down Cake

*Don Mauer*

SERVES 15

DON MAUER'S GREAT-GRANDMOTHER was known for a much higher-fat version of this unique cake. Spoon the "gooey" fudge, which sinks to the bottom during the baking, over each piece of cake, and top with a dab of reduced-fat whipped topping or vanilla frozen yogurt. This recipe was adapted slightly from one in Don Mauer's *Lean and Lovin' It* (Chapters Publishing).

CAKE

2 cups all-purpose flour
¼ cup unsweetened cocoa powder
4 teaspoons baking powder
1⅔ cups granulated sugar
1 cup skim milk, room temperature
¼ cup nonfat plain yogurt
2 teaspoons vanilla extract
1 ounce unsweetened chocolate, melted and cooled slightly

SAUCE

1 cup granulated sugar
1 cup firmly packed dark brown sugar
½ cup plus 2 tablespoons unsweetened cocoa powder
1¾ cups hot water

1. Preheat oven to 325 degrees F, with a rack in center. Lightly spray bottom and sides of a 9-x-13-inch glass baking dish with nonstick cooking spray; set aside.

2. **To make cake:** In a medium bowl, sift together flour, cocoa powder and baking powder. Set aside.

3. In a large mixing bowl, whisk together sugar, milk, yogurt, vanilla and chocolate until combined, about 1 minute. Add sifted ingredients and whisk until just moistened, 30 to 40 seconds.

4. Pour batter into prepared baking dish and smooth top. Set aside while preparing sauce.

5. **To make sauce**: In a medium bowl, whisk together both sugars and cocoa. Gradually add water and whisk until sugar is dissolved and sauce is smooth, about 30 seconds.

6. Gently pour sauce over back of a spoon or a rubber spatula to drizzle onto cake batter, covering completely. (If some batter floats up from bottom, do not be concerned.) Bake until cake is firm to the touch, 45 to 50 minutes. Let cool in pan for about 30 minutes.

7. Cut warm cake into 15 squares. Transfer squares to plates. Spoon fudge sauce from bottom of baking dish over cake and serve warm, or if you prefer, chill before serving. (Don notes that this cake can be cooled, covered and kept for about 2 days.)

PER SERVING: CALORIES: 284; FAT: 2 G; CHOLESTEROL: 0 MG; SODIUM: 149 MG; PROTEIN: 4 G; CARBOHYDRATE: 67 G

# Rich Chocolate Cake with Raspberry Sauce

*Cathy B.*

SERVES 12

**T**HIS IS A GREAT MAKE-AHEAD PARTY CAKE, because it's best kept in the refrigerator for at least one night and served cold. It's rich, chocolaty and velvety. (If you don't want to make your own sauce, you can substitute raspberry preserves, heated and thinned with a little water, then cooled for 15 minutes.) Garnish Cathy's cake with fresh mint leaves and/or a sprinkling of shaved chocolate.

CAKE

1¾  cups all-purpose flour
2  cups granulated sugar
¾  cup cocoa powder
1½  teaspoons baking soda
1  teaspoon salt
2  large egg whites
1  cup skim milk
½  cup canned pumpkin (for pie)
1  tablespoon vanilla extract
1  cup water, heated to boiling

SAUCE

1  cup fresh raspberries, plus 10 whole berries
   for garnish (or substitute partially thawed
   frozen berries, without added sugar)
¼  cup granulated sugar
1  ounce (2 tablespoons) kirsch liqueur

1. Preheat oven to 350 degrees F, with a rack in center. Spray two 8-inch round pans with nonstick cooking spray; dust each with a small amount of flour. Shake any excess flour from pans; set aside.

2. **To make cake:** In a medium bowl, sift together flour, sugar, cocoa powder, baking soda and salt. Set aside. In a large mixing bowl, whisk together egg whites, milk, pumpkin and vanilla.

3. Add liquid ingredients to dry ingredients and mix with an electric mixer on low speed until ingredients are moistened. Beat on medium speed for 2 minutes. With mixer on low speed, slowly add water, mixing until batter is smooth.

4. Pour into prepared pans. Bake for 35 to 40 minutes, or until a toothpick inserted in center of cakes comes out clean. Cool slightly; remove from pans.

5. **To make sauce:** Puree 1 cup berries, sugar and kirsch in a blender or food processor. If desired, strain sauce and chill until ready to use.

6. When cake is cool, slice rounds in half horizontally and spread about ¼ cup raspberry sauce evenly over three of the layers. Stack one layer on top of another. On the fourth and top layer, spread remaining sauce (you will have about ½ cup) and dot evenly with whole raspberries.

PER SERVING: CALORIES: 256; FAT: 1 G; CHOLESTEROL: 0 MG; SODIUM: 358 MG; PROTEIN: 4 G; CARBOHYDRATE: 59 G

# Raisin-Spice Layer Cake

*Joy C.*

SERVES 10 TO 12

**M**Y HUSBAND, the world's greatest lover of spice cake, gave top marks to this moist, flavorful version. You can also make it like a sheet cake, in a jellyroll pan. The cake freezes well.

CAKE

| | |
|---|---|
| 2 | cups water |
| 1 | cup dark raisins |
| ¼ | cup margarine |
| 1 | jar (4 ounces) baby food applesauce |
| 3 | cups all-purpose flour |
| 1½ | cups granulated sugar |
| 2 | teaspoons baking powder |
| 2 | teaspoons baking soda |
| 2 | teaspoons ground cinnamon |
| 1 | teaspoon ground nutmeg |
| ½ | teaspoon ground cloves |
| ½ | teaspoon ground allspice |

OPTIONAL CREAM CHEESE FROSTING

| | |
|---|---|
| 3 | cups powdered sugar |
| ¼ | cup Neufchâtel cheese, room temperature |
| 2 | tablespoons evaporated skim milk |
| 1 | teaspoon maple flavoring or vanilla extract |
| 2 | tablespoons walnuts, chopped (½ ounce) |

1. Preheat oven to 350 degrees F, with a rack in center. Spray two 8-inch round pans with nonstick cooking spray. Set aside.

2. **To make cake:** Bring water, raisins and margarine to a boil in a medium saucepan. Remove from heat. Stir in applesauce; set aside.

3. In a large bowl, stir together flour, sugar, baking powder, baking soda, cinnamon, nutmeg, cloves and allspice.

4. With a wooden spoon, gently stir raisin mixture into dry ingredients until well blended; do not overmix.

5. Pour batter into prepared pans, dividing evenly and smoothing. Bake for 30 minutes, or until a toothpick inserted in center comes out clean.

6. **To make optional frosting:** In a medium bowl, with a wooden spoon or an electric mixer, beat powdered sugar, Neufchâtel, milk and maple flavoring or vanilla until smooth.

7. When cake is cool, spread frosting on top and drizzle sides. Sprinkle walnuts over top.

PER SERVING WITHOUT FROSTING: CALORIES: 295; FAT: 4 G; CHOLESTEROL: 0 MG; SODIUM: 341 MG; PROTEIN: 4 G; CARBOHYDRATE: 62 G

PER SERVING WITH FROSTING: CALORIES: 435; FAT: 6 G; CHOLESTEROL: 4 MG; SODIUM: 363 MG; PROTEIN: 5 G; CARBOHYDRATE: 93 G

# Jamaican Banana Cake

*Cathy B.*

SERVES 15

A PERFECT WAY to use up overripe bananas and, at the same time, indulge in a fat-free dessert. Serve for dessert or for breakfast. Cathy likes to serve it with Tropical Fruit Sauce (page 334).

- 3   large egg whites
- ½   teaspoon apple cider vinegar
- 1¼   cups granulated sugar
- 1¾   cups sifted all-purpose flour
- 2   teaspoons baking powder
- ½   teaspoon baking soda
- ½   teaspoon ground allspice
- ½   teaspoon ground nutmeg
- 2   cups mashed very ripe banana
  (about 4 medium or about 1½ pounds before peeling)
- 1   ounce rum or 1 teaspoon rum extract
- 1   teaspoon vanilla extract
- ⅓   cup skim milk

1. Preheat oven to 350 degrees F, with a rack in center. Spray a 9-x-13-inch cake pan with nonstick cooking spray. Set aside.

2. With an electric mixer on high speed, beat egg whites with vinegar, slowly adding ¼ cup sugar. Beat until stiff peaks form; set aside.

3. In a medium bowl, sift together flour, baking powder, baking soda, allspice and nutmeg. Set aside.

4. In a large bowl, with a wooden spoon, stir together banana, rum or rum extract, vanilla and remaining 1 cup sugar. Add dry ingredients to banana mixture alternately with milk, mixing with a wooden spoon or a rubber spatula until ingredients are just combined.

5. Gently fold in egg whites. Pour batter into prepared pan. Bake for 25 to 30 minutes, or until a toothpick inserted in center of cake comes out clean. Cool in pan. Cut into 15 pieces and serve at room temperature. Cake can be stored in pan, covered tightly with foil. (Refrigerate if not eating within 2 to 3 days.)

PER SERVING: CALORIES: 152; FAT: 0 G; CHOLESTEROL: 0 MG; SODIUM: 121 MG; PROTEIN: 3 G; CARBOHYDRATE: 35 G

# Crème de Menthe Cheesecake

*Catherine C.*

SERVES 6 TO 8

THIS PRETTY, MINTY CHEESECAKE, meant for company, is complemented by freshly brewed coffee.

CHEESECAKE

¼ cup crushed chocolate wafer crumbs (about 4)
1 cup 1% cottage cheese
1 package (8 ounces) Neufchâtel cheese
¾ cup granulated sugar
2 tablespoons all-purpose flour
2 large eggs or ½ cup egg substitute, thawed
¼ cup crème de menthe liqueur

CHOCOLATE TOPPING

¼ cup granulated sugar
3 tablespoons cocoa powder
1 teaspoon cornstarch
7 tablespoons water
½ teaspoon vanilla extract

1. Preheat oven to 300 degrees F, with a rack in center. Spray a 9-inch springform pan with nonstick cooking spray.

2. **To make cheesecake:** Sprinkle wafer crumbs in bottom of pan and gently shake to coat bottom evenly; set aside.

3. In a food processor fitted with the metal blade, combine cottage cheese, Neufchâtel, sugar, flour, eggs or egg substitute and crème de menthe. Process until very smooth. Spoon into prepared pan and smooth top with a rubber spatula.

4. Bake until set in center, 35 to 40 minutes. Cool in pan. Refrigerate until cold, 2 to 3 hours. Loosen sides of cake with a small spatula or knife and remove pan rim.

5. **Meanwhile, make topping:** In a small saucepan, combine sugar, cocoa powder and cornstarch. Add water slowly, stirring. Cook over medium heat, stirring constantly, until sauce has thickened, 3 to 5 minutes. Cook for 1 minute longer, continuing to stir. Remove from heat and add vanilla. Chill until cool to the touch.

6. Spread topping evenly over top of cheesecake. Serve immediately or refrigerate and serve later.

PER SERVING: CALORIES: 267; FAT: 9 G; CHOLESTEROL: 76 MG; SODIUM: 265 MG;

PROTEIN: 9 G; CARBOHYDRATE: 36 G

# Chocolate Amaretto Cheesecake

*Beth W.*

SERVES 6 TO 8

FOR A TREAT, top this rich cheesecake with the mocha version of Vanilla Frozen Custard (page 338).

⅓ cup crushed chocolate wafers (about 6)
1½ cups fat-free cream cheese (about 12 ounces)
½ cup granulated sugar
1 packet Sweet 'N Low
1 cup nonfat cottage cheese
1 large egg
¼ cup unsweetened cocoa powder
¼ cup all-purpose flour
¼ cup amaretto liqueur
1 teaspoon vanilla extract
2 tablespoons mini-chocolate chips

1. Preheat oven to 300 degrees F, with a rack in center. Spray a 9- or 10-inch springform pan with nonstick cooking spray. Sprinkle wafer crumbs evenly over bottom of pan; set aside.

2. Place cream cheese, sugar, sweetener, cottage cheese, egg, cocoa powder, flour, amaretto and vanilla in a food processor fitted with the metal blade, or a blender, and process until smooth, about 1 minute. Pour into a bowl and fold in chocolate chips.

3. Slowly pour batter over crumbs in prepared pan. Bake until cheesecake is set, 50 to 55 minutes. Cool completely on a wire rack. Loosen sides of cake with a small spatula or knife and remove pan rim. Cover with plastic wrap and chill, preferably for at least 8 hours, before serving.

PER SERVING: CALORIES: 204; FAT: 2.5 G; CHOLESTEROL: 35 MG; SODIUM: 338 MG; PROTEIN: 14 G; CARBOHYDRATE: 30 G

# Southern Banana-Butterscotch Cream Pie

*JoAnna M. Lund*

SERVES 6 TO 8

JOANNA CAME UP WITH THIS simple low-fat pie for her daughter when she came home for a visit. The creamy combination of butterscotch pudding, banana and maple syrup is luscious. This recipe was adapted from one in JoAnna Lund's *Healthy Exchanges Cookbook* (G.P. Putnam's Sons).

1 package (4-serving) sugar-free instant butterscotch pudding mix
⅔ cup nonfat dry milk powder
1 cup water
¼ cup reduced-calorie maple syrup
¾ cup thawed low-calorie whipped topping
2 ripe medium bananas (11-12 ounces)
1 graham cracker pie crust (6 ounces; look for brand with lowest fat level)
2 tablespoons chopped pecans (½ ounce)

1. In a medium bowl, combine pudding mix and milk powder; set aside.

2. In a small bowl, whisk together water, maple syrup and ¼ cup whipped topping until blended. With a wire whisk, add liquid mixture to dry pudding mixture and whisk until well blended. Set aside.

3. Peel and slice bananas, evenly distributing them over pie crust. Spoon pudding mixture over bananas.

4. Spread remaining ½ cup whipped topping over pudding and sprinkle with pecans. Chill before serving.

PER SERVING: CALORIES: 220; FAT: 8 G; CHOLESTEROL: 0 MG; SODIUM: 346 MG;

PROTEIN: 5 G; CARBOHYDRATE: 34 G

# Deep-Dish Pumpkin Pie

*Virginia L.*

SERVES 6 TO 8

**V**IRGINIA PUTS A NEW SPIN ON PUMPKIN PIE by adding maple flavoring and using a graham cracker crust. Because she is lactose-intolerant, she uses nondairy creamer in place of evaporated milk. The crust is crunchy when first made but becomes soft and cakelike after a few days, and the flavor pleasantly intensifies.

CRUST
6   whole graham crackers (12 squares),
    rolled into crumbs
½   cup all-purpose flour
½   cup whole wheat flour
⅓   cup (5⅓ tablespoons) diet margarine, melted
¼   cup firmly packed dark brown sugar
2   tablespoons granulated sugar

FILLING
1   can (15 ounces) pumpkin (for pie)
1½  cups evaporated skim milk
    or fat-free nondairy creamer
½   cup (4-ounce carton) egg substitute,
    thawed, or 2 large eggs
½   cup firmly packed dark brown sugar
1   tablespoon all-purpose flour
2   teaspoons maple flavoring
1   teaspoon ground cinnamon
½   teaspoon ground nutmeg
¼   teaspoon salt

1. Preheat oven to 450 degrees F, with a rack in center. Spray a 10-inch deep-dish pie pan with nonstick spray. Set aside.

2. **To make crust:** Mix all ingredients by hand until well combined. Pat gently and evenly into bottom and up sides of prepared pan. (Don't press too firmly.) Set aside.

3. **To make filling:** In a large bowl, whisk together all ingredients until thoroughly combined. Pour into pie crust.

4. Bake for 15 minutes; reduce oven temperature to 350 degrees and bake for about 30 minutes, or until firm in center and a knife inserted in center comes out clean. Cool completely on a wire rack before serving.

PER SERVING: CALORIES: 298; FAT: 6 G; CHOLESTEROL: 0 MG; SODIUM: 316 MG; PROTEIN: 9 G; CARBOHYDRATE: 55 G

# No-Guilt Chocolate Cream Pie

*Mary Ann K.*

SERVES 6 TO 8

THIS EXTRA-EASY CHOCOLATE CREAM PIE gets some vanilla yogurt folded in at the end. Top with reduced-fat whipped topping.

PIE CRUST

1½ cups graham cracker crumbs
(about 10 full-sized crackers)
1 tablespoon granulated sugar
4 tablespoons (½ stick) diet margarine, melted

FILLING

1 package (4-serving) sugar-free regular
chocolate pudding mix (not instant)
1½ cups cold skim milk
3 tablespoons nonfat dry milk powder
½ cup nonfat vanilla yogurt

1. Preheat oven to 350 degrees F, with a rack in center.

2. **To make pie crust:** In a 9-inch pie pan, mix graham cracker crumbs and sugar; stir in melted margarine. With your hands, press mixture evenly into bottom of pan. Bake for 15 minutes, or until it begins to brown. Remove from oven and cool completely; set aside.

3. **To make filling:** Cook pudding mix according to package directions, but use 1½ cups skim milk instead of recommended amount. While it is still warm, whisk in milk powder. Cool to room temperature.

4. Fold in vanilla yogurt. Spread over graham cracker crust, and refrigerate for 3 hours, or until firm. Serve cold.

PER SERVING: CALORIES: 150; FAT: 5 G; CHOLESTEROL: 0 MG; SODIUM: 271 MG;
PROTEIN: 5 G; CARBOHYDRATE: 23 G

# Strawberry Sauce

*Diane J.*

MAKES 1¼ CUPS OR 5 SERVINGS, EACH ¼ CUP

A TOUCH OF GINGER gives this sauce an exquisite taste. Diane likes to serve it over fresh fruit, such as fresh pineapple mixed with strawberries. But it is also good mixed into plain yogurt or spooned over angel food cake, sherbet or vanilla frozen yogurt.

1    package (10 ounces) frozen unsweetened
      strawberries, slightly thawed
5    packages low-calorie sweetener, such as Equal
1½   teaspoons fresh lime juice
1    piece gingerroot (1 x ½ inch), peeled

1. Place all ingredients in a blender or a food processor fitted with the metal blade and blend until smooth.

2. Refrigerate for 1 hour before serving, to let flavors blend.

PER SERVING: CALORIES: 26; FAT: 0 G; CHOLESTEROL: 0 MG; SODIUM: 1 MG; PROTEIN: 0 G; CARBOHYDRATE: 7 G

# Tropical Fruit Sauce

*Cathy B.*

MAKES ABOUT 2 CUPS OR 8 SERVINGS, EACH ¼ CUP

THIS SWEET AND TART SAUCE complements unfrosted low-fat cakes, such as angel food, Orange Delight Pound Cake (page 317) and Jamaican Banana Cake (page 324). It's a good topping for vanilla frozen yogurt or mixed into plain yogurt.

    8   ounces fresh pineapple (about ½ fresh pineapple),
        peeled and cored
    1   medium papaya (about 14 ounces),
        peeled and seeded
    ½   cup fresh lemon juice (3 medium lemons)
    1   cup granulated sugar

1. Cut pineapple and papaya into small pieces. Puree in a blender or a food processor fitted with the metal blade.

2. Pour into a medium nonaluminum saucepan. Add lemon juice and sugar. Bring to a boil over high heat, stirring often. Lower heat and simmer until sauce coats a spoon, about 20 minutes. Chill before serving.

PER SERVING: CALORIES: 129; FAT: 0 G; CHOLESTEROL: 0 MG; SODIUM: 2 MG; PROTEIN: 0 G; CARBOHYDRATE: 34 G

# Pudding Fruit Parfait

*Ann F.*

SERVES 4

NOTHING COULD BE EASIER—and prettier—than fruit layered with creamy pudding. Just before serving, top this refreshing dessert with a tablespoon of reduced-fat whipped topping, a dash of cinnamon and a vanilla wafer.

1 large peach, peeled and thinly sliced (about 1 cup)
2 cups sugar-free regular vanilla pudding (not instant), made according to package directions, using skim milk
1 cup fresh blueberries
6 medium strawberries, sliced (about 1 cup)

In 4 large stemmed goblets or parfait dishes, divide and layer fruit and pudding as follows: all of peach slices, one-third of pudding, all of blueberries, one-third of pudding, all of strawberry slices and remaining one-third of pudding. Serve immediately, or chill for 30 to 60 minutes. This is best if served within 2 hours.

PER SERVING: CALORIES: 155; FAT: 0.5 G; CHOLESTEROL: 0 MG; SODIUM: 422 MG; PROTEIN: 5 G; CARBOHYDRATE: 34 G

# Quick Raspberry Sherbet

## *Diane J.*

MAKES APPROXIMATELY 2 CUPS OR 4 SERVINGS

A N ATTRACTIVE DEEP ROSY PINK, Diane's refreshing soft sherbet is a perfect ending to a heavy or spicy meal. It's so simple that it can be made at a moment's notice. In place of raspberries, Diane says you can use frozen blueberries, strawberries or any mixture of frozen fruit you like.

3  cups frozen unsweetened raspberries
    (12-ounce bag), thawed slightly
¼  cup granulated sugar
¼  cup water, or more as needed
2  tablespoons nonfat dry milk powder
2  packets low-calorie sweetener, such as Equal
2  teaspoons vanilla extract

1. Place all ingredients in a blender or a food processor fitted with the metal blade.

2. Blend until mixture is the consistency of soft sherbet. You may need to add more water, ½ teaspoon at a time, if sherbet is too thick. Serve immediately. (If you make sherbet ahead and freeze it, soften before serving by letting it sit at room temperature or by defrosting in microwave for a short time.)

PER SERVING: CALORIES: 105; FAT: 0 G; CHOLESTEROL: 0 MG; SODIUM: 21 MG; PROTEIN: 2 G; CARBOHYDRATE: 24 G

# Peach-Almond Sorbet

*Diane J.*

MAKES APPROXIMATELY 3 CUPS OR 6 SERVINGS

THIS LIGHT AND REFRESHING FAT-FREE FROZEN DESSERT is perfect after a filling meal or as a treat on a hot summer afternoon. Diane likes to garnish each serving with a small amount of shredded coconut.

1   package (16 ounces) frozen sliced peaches
¾   cup water
¼   cup Tang powder
¼   cup granulated sugar
1   packet low-calorie sweetener, such as Equal
½   teaspoon almond extract

Place all ingredients in a blender or a food processor fitted with the metal blade. Blend until smooth, about 1 minute. Serve immediately. (Sorbet will be soft.)

PER SERVING: CALORIES: 136; FAT: 0 G; CHOLESTEROL: 0 MG; SODIUM: 7 MG; PROTEIN: 0 G; CARBOHYDRATE: 35 G

# Vanilla Frozen Custard

*Catherine C.*

MAKES ABOUT 3 CUPS OR 6 SERVINGS

YOU'LL NEED AN ICE CREAM FREEZER for this one. It can be made using a microwave oven or on top of the stove. Enjoy the creamy vanilla version, or try one of Catherine's variations. (If you like coffee ice cream, the mocha version is outstanding.) This ice cream is best served soft.

    1½   cups 1% milk
    ¼    cup granulated sugar
    1    tablespoon all-purpose flour
    ½    cup (4-ounce carton) egg substitute, thawed
    1½   cups thawed reduced-fat frozen whipped topping
    2    teaspoons vanilla extract

Microwave method:

1. Pour milk into a large microwavable bowl, and heat on high power for 2 minutes.

2. Meanwhile, mix sugar and flour in a small bowl. Whisk into hot milk. Return milk mixture to microwave and cook on high power for 2 minutes. Thoroughly stir and cook for 2 minutes more on high. Repeat once more.

3. Put egg substitute into a small heatproof bowl. Stirring constantly, slowly pour 1 cup hot milk mixture into egg substitute. Pour warmed egg mixture back into hot milk mixture and stir thoroughly.

4. Return mixture to microwave and cook on high power for 1 minute. Stir and cook once more on high power for about 1 minute, or until mixture is thick and looks like custard. Cover with plastic wrap and refrigerate for at least 4 hours.

**Stovetop method:** In a medium saucepan, heat milk until warm to the touch. Mix sugar and flour; whisk into warm milk. Bring to a boil, stirring often. Whisk 1 cup hot milk into egg substitute in a small heatproof bowl; pour warmed egg mixture back into saucepan. Over medium-high heat, cook for 1 to 2 minutes, or until mixture is thick and looks like custard, stirring constantly. Remove from heat, pour into a bowl, cover with plastic wrap and refrigerate for at least 4 hours.

5. Just before freezing in an ice cream freezer, fold whipped topping and vanilla into custard mixture.

6. Freeze according to manufacturer's instructions. Custard is best served immediately. (If you keep it in the freezer, you can soften it by letting it sit at room temperature or microwaving on defrost for a short time.)

PER SERVING: CALORIES: 123; FAT: 4 G; CHOLESTEROL: 3 MG; SODIUM: 73 MG; PROTEIN: 5 G; CARBOHYDRATE: 17 G

### Variations

**Fruit:** Mash 1 cup of your favorite fruit, such as strawberries or bananas, and add with whipped topping and vanilla in step 5. Continue as directed.

**Mocha:** Add 1 teaspoon instant coffee plus 1 tablespoon cocoa powder to flour and sugar mixture before adding to milk. Continue as directed.

# Peach Shake

*Catherine C.*

MAKES APPROXIMATELY 3 SERVINGS, EACH 1 CUP

THIS FAT-FREE SHAKE is the perfect beverage for a hot summer day. It also makes a nice nonalcoholic drink for a cocktail party selection. Serve it in a frosted mug or stemware glass, and garnish with a sprig of fresh mint.

|     |                                                              |
| --- | ------------------------------------------------------------ |
| 1   | cup peeled, pitted and sliced fresh or canned peaches or nectarines |
| ¾   | cup peach nectar                                             |
| ¾   | cup nonfat frozen yogurt or nonfat ice milk (vanilla or any fruit flavor) |
| ⅓   | cup nonfat dry milk powder                                   |
| 1   | ice cube                                                     |

Place all ingredients in a blender or a food processor fitted with the metal blade. Cover tightly and blend until thick and creamy. It is best if served immediately but keeps in the refrigerator for several hours; you may want to whir it again before serving.

PER SERVING: CALORIES: 143; FAT: 0 G; CHOLESTEROL: 3 MG; SODIUM: 99 MG; PROTEIN: 8 G; CARBOHYDRATE: 29 G

# Strawberry-Cranberry Frappé

*Catherine C.*

MAKES APPROXIMATELY 2 SERVINGS, EACH 1 CUP

TO TURN THIS FRAPPÉ into a sherbetlike dessert, use frozen instead of fresh strawberries.

1 cup fresh strawberries, sliced
¾ cup vanilla or strawberry nonfat yogurt
   or nonfat ice milk
¾ cup reduced-calorie cranberry juice cocktail
¼ cup nonfat dry milk powder

Place all ingredients in a blender or a food processor fitted with the metal blade. Cover tightly and blend until thick and smooth. (Strain if you dislike seeds.) Frappé is best served immediately but keeps in refrigerator for several hours; you may want to whir it again before serving.

PER SERVING: CALORIES: 150; FAT: 0 G; CHOLESTEROL: 3 MG; SODIUM: 119 MG;

PROTEIN: 9 G; CARBOHYDRATE: 28 G

# Banana-Strawberry Smoothie

*Mary Ann K.*

MAKES APPROXIMATELY 4 SERVINGS, EACH 1 CUP

WHEN YOU HAVE OVERRIPE BANANAS, just peel them, pop them into a plastic bag and freeze so you're always ready to throw together one of Mary Ann's favorite snacks. The frozen bananas give this smoothie a thick, creamy texture.

2   very ripe medium bananas (11-12 ounces), peeled, frozen and broken into 4-5 segments
8   large strawberries
1½  cups skim milk
1-2  packets low-calorie sweetener, such as Equal
1   teaspoon vanilla extract

Place all ingredients in a blender or a food processor fitted with the metal blade and blend until smooth. Serve immediately in frosty mugs.

PER SERVING: CALORIES: 104; FAT: 0.5 G; CHOLESTEROL: 0 MG; SODIUM: 48 MG; PROTEIN: 4 G; CARBOHYDRATE: 22 G

# INDEX

and menstruation, 85-86
overeating, 49
at parties, 105-6
and planned meals, 50-53
protein for fullness feeling, 33-34
and regular meals, 61-62
in restaurants, 98-104
slower, 53
at tough time of day, 84-85
on vacation, 106-7
Egg(s)
Deviled, Blue Cheese, 199
Drop Chicken Soup, 196
Salad, Mock, Sandwich, 183
Eggplant Soufflé, 292
exercise
and food balance, 139
and maintenance, 139
and smoking, 91-92

Fajitas, Cilantro-Veggie, 201
family eating habits and weight control,
96-97
fast food, 98, 101
fast food choices in restaurants, 102
fat. *See also* low-fat
added, 36-37
calories in, 35
claims on food labels, 58
desire for, 37-38
and food satisfaction, 33
-free foods, 38, 58, 59
gram allowance, daily, 35
intake, recording, 32-33
negligible, in meal plan, 113
recommendations for, in diet, 57
-reduced cooking, 144-46
saving, in restaurants, 102-4
storing, in body, 36
fiber in the diet, 33, 43
fiber intake, boosting, 43

Fish
Cheddar, 229
in the diet, 44, 57
Pirate's Pie, 230
food(s)
buddies, 89-90
cravings, 66-67, 69-72, 75, 85-86
diary, keeping, 138-39
Food Guide Pyramid, 56
forbidden, 65-67. *See also* tempting
foods
free, in weight-loss plan, 136
fullness from, 33
good/bad, thinking about, 65-66
groups, recommended daily
servings from, 56-57
labels, 58
learning about, 32-33
pushers, 82-83, 86-88
tempting, 63-72, 75, 138
Frappé, Strawberry-Cranberry, 341. *See
also* Frozen Dessert
free (calorie) foods, 136
French Bread Croutons, 270
French Fries, Mike's, 299
friends, changes in, with weight loss,
89-91
Frosting, Chocolate, Rich, 310
Frozen Custard, Vanilla, 338;
variations, 339
Frozen Dessert
Peach-Almond Sorbet, 337
Raspberry Sherbet, Quick, 336
Strawberry-Cranberry Frappé, 341
Vanilla Frozen Custard, 338;
variations, 339
Fruit(s)
eating for weight control, 40
Fruity Bread Pudding, 306
and Greens in Raspberry
Vinaigrette, 283
-Molasses Bars, 312
Parfait, Pudding, 335